SUPER SIMPLE

ANATOMY & PHYSIOLOGY

LABORATORY MANUAL

SUPER SIMPLE

ANATOMY & PHYSIOLOGY

LABORATORY MANUAL

SECOND EDITION

Nelson H. Kraus

Ivy Tech Community College

cognella
SAN DIEGO

Bassim Hamadeh, CEO and Publisher
Carrie Baarns, Senior Manager, Revisions and Author Care
Kaela Martin, Project Editor
Susana Christie, Senior Developmental Editor
Laureen Gleason, Production Editor
Jess Estrella, Senior Graphic Designer
Trey Soto, Licensing Specialist
Jaye Pratt, Interior Designer
Natalie Piccotti, Director of Marketing
Kassie Graves, Senior Vice President of Editorial
Jamie Giganti, Director of Academic Publishing

Printed in the United States of America.

cognella® ACADEMIC PUBLISHING
3970 Sorrento Valley Blvd., Ste. 500, San Diego, CA 92121

CONTENTS

INTRODUCTION

THE ULTIMATE STUDY TOOL

Welcome to a unique and highly effective series of simple activities that utilize neuroscientifically proven techniques to facilitate student understanding of anatomy and physiology.

This lab manual is designed to augment any reference text in an introductory human anatomy and physiology course. More specifically, it is focused to complement the 2nd Edition of the *Super Simple Anatomy and Physiology* text (Cognella, 2021).

The *SS A&P Lab Manual* allows students to revisit and review material already covered in a lecture/discussion class setting. There is evolving neuroscientific evidence to demonstrate the importance of engaging students in activities to facilitate learning and deepen understanding. The *SS A&P Lab Manual* provides students an opportunity to learn by creating, drawing, coloring, researching, and discussing both human structure and function.

The manual is organized into thirty-two activities that parallel the twenty-one chapters in the *SS A&P* text, 2nd Edition. Activities start with "A&P Basics" covering nomenclature, terms, planes, regions, body cavities, abdominal quadrants, and body regions. It then moves through "Chemistry Basics," "Energy Production," "Protein Synthesis," and "Simplified Cell Biology." The remaining activities cover topics from histology, muscles, the nervous system, the cardiovascular system (CVS), through the reproductive system, fluids and electrolytes, and acid/base balance.

The lab manual contains more activities than can be accomplished in a one-semester or even a two-semester introductory A&P course. Individual anatomy or physiology courses can "pick and choose" those activities most helpful. Instructors (and students) are encouraged to select those activities that are most relevant for each individual class. This will depend on the length of the course; whether the course combines A&P or is focused on A&P individually; whether it is delivered in person, virtually, or in a hybrid format; and facility or institutional limitations. The *SS A&P Lab Manual* is designed to be flexible so it will fit a wide diversity of settings.

Each activity is designed in a similar fashion to take advantage of the kinesthetic power of actively researching, drawing, and coloring structures, functions, and concepts. All activities start with a brief description of the purpose of the lab. This is followed by an individual pre-lab worksheet (perforated so students can tear it out) that can be collected at the beginning of an in-person lab or submitted electronically in a virtual setting. The pre-lab worksheet incentivizes students to prepare *before* the lab session.

Activities to be accomplished during the lab are then described involving researching, creating, drawing, and coloring graphics of structures and functions. This is followed by a random selection of a lab "team" (a roll of the dice) who will lead a class discussion of their graphics by asking and answering questions of their classmates (peer instruction). This process takes advantage of the fact that in *any* learning environment, the ones doing the most work are the ones doing the most learning!

Finally, each activity has a lab team worksheet, which is completed by lab teams during the lab session. These are turned in at the end of the lab and encourage team discussion of the topic. The consistent format of all activities eliminates confusion and the need for repetitive instructor explanation. This maximizes time for student engagement and learning.

Some (but not all) of the Lab Activities have images depicting the concept covered or providing an opportunity for students to "practice" the material. The application and utilization of those images allow instructors to help deepen student insight. The images not only tell a "story" about basic anatomy and physiology but provide coloring and labeling opportunities for the students. Students are encouraged to complete Lab activities on their own, whether assigned or not.

This manual is just like any piece of exercise equipment.

You've got to *use it* to benefit!

Let's ride!

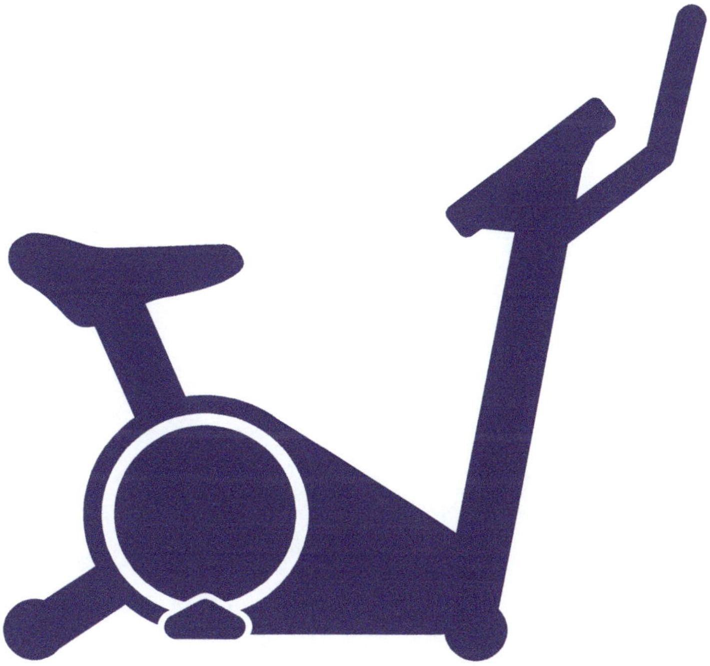

LAB 1

A&P Basics: Nomenclature through Body Regions

Purpose of Lab and Desired Outcomes

Participate in Individual and Lab Team Activities to gain insight and understanding into the following topics:

1. Definitions of A&P
2. Basic anatomical terms and nomenclature
3. Abdominal quadrants and abdominal regions
4. Open and closed body cavities
5. Membranes and mesentery
6. Anatomical regions
7. Anatomical planes
8. Basic concept of anatomy and physiology
9. Anatomical position

Pre-Lab Worksheet

LAB 1—ESSENTIAL "STUFF" YOU NEED TO KNOW

Name: **Date:**

Each student should answer the following questions *before* coming to Lab.

Complete the pre-lab reading assignments for this Lab Activity. Then, answer the following questions:

1. Anatomy is the study of human ________________.
2. Physiology is the study of human ________________.
3. Anterior is the same as ____________ or the ____________ of the body.
4. A ____________ plane divides the body into unequal left and right sections.
5. A ____________ plane divides the body into superior and inferior sections.
6. The serous membrane that supports the small intestines is called the ____________.
7. Closed body cavities are lined by ____________ membranes.
8. Open body cavities are lined by ____________ membranes.
9. The ____________ plane divides the body into anterior and posterior sections.

In-Lab Activities

1. Collection of student Pre-Lab Worksheets.
2. Instructor calls for QCs (Student Questions, Concerns, Confusions, and need for Clarification) and class discusses QCs.
3. Brief instructor explanation of In-Lab Activities and desired outcomes from Lab time.
4. Lab Teams will write out the "Body Cavities Flow Chart" shown in Figure 4.3 in *SS A&P*, 2nd Edition. Or Teams will produce a graphic presentation (PPTs, Prezi, or Google Slides) in a virtual environment.
5. Lab Teams will draw and label as many body regions as possible in the time allotted or produce a graphic presentation (PPTs, Prezi, or Google Slides) in a virtual environment.
    - Discuss the graphic among Team members.
    - Ask each other questions.
    - Teach each other.
    - Prepare a verbal explanation of the graphic.
    - Be prepared to share the graphic and lead a discussion with the entire Lab.
    - Teams complete the Team Lab Worksheet for turning in at the end of Lab.
6. A randomly selected Lab Team will lead a class discussion of their body regions graphic with the entire class by *engaging the rest of the class* in a *discussion* of body regions by asking colleagues questions. This is a discussion and not a presentation.
    - Teams will be prepared to do Q&A with students and instructor.
    - Each Team will take a picture of their final body regions graphic and electronically submit it to instructor/TA.
    - Each Team will turn in one Team Worksheet to instructor/TA.
7. Instructor will complete "Major Takeaways" with the class.

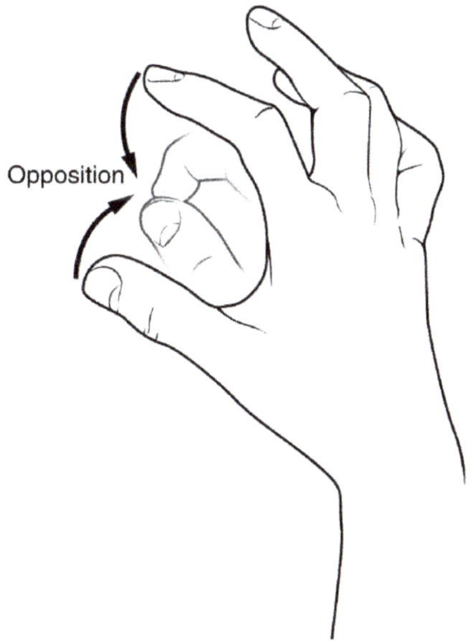

FIGURE 1.1 The human hand can oppose because of the way it's structured.

Opposition—placing the thumb against the fingers sets the human apart.

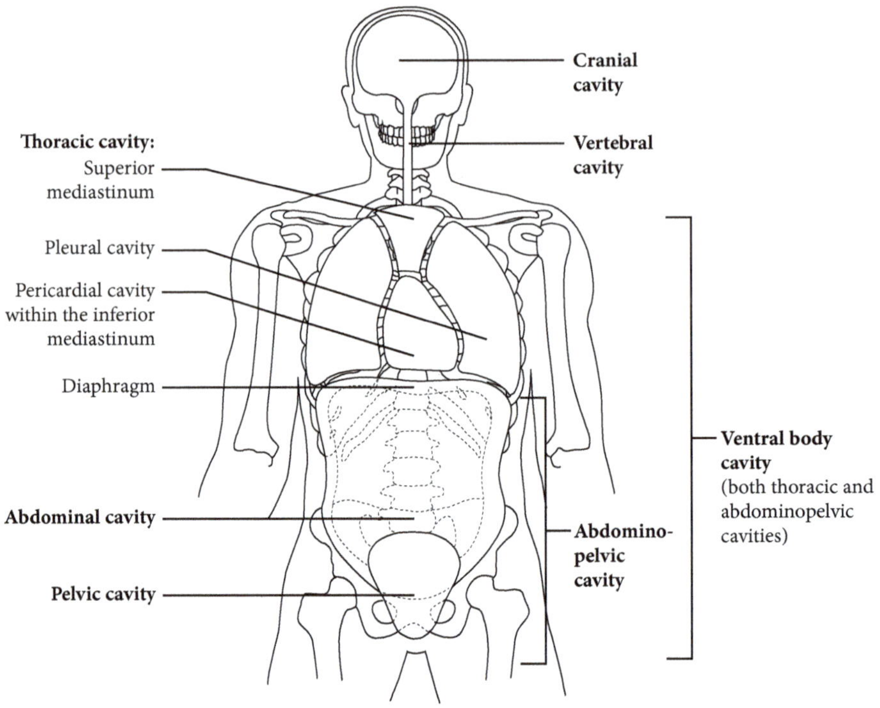

FIGURE 1.2A Closed body cavities are divided into dorsal and ventral. Color them different colors.

Closed body cavities contain viscera and are lined by serous membranes, which produce a thin, watery fluid providing lubrication.

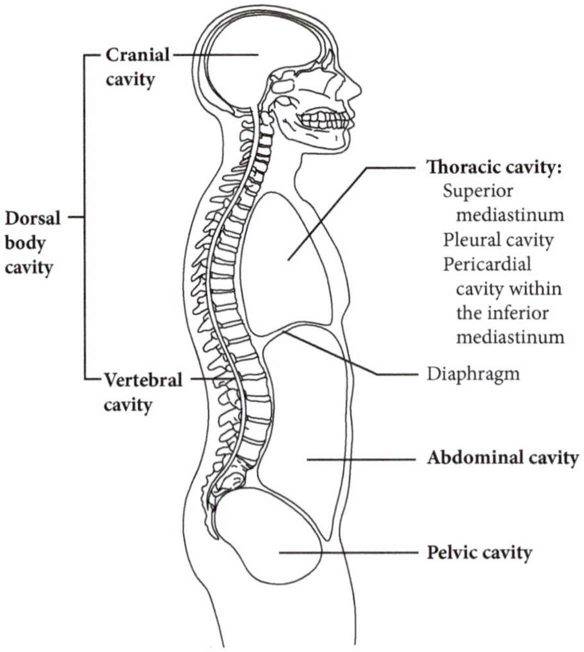

FIGURE 1.2B Closed body cavities are divided into dorsal and ventral. Color them different colors.

What structure separates the thoracic cavity from the abdominopelvic cavity?

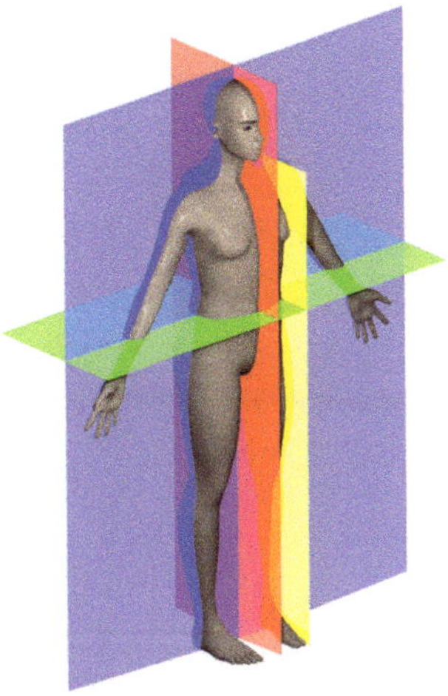

FIGURE 1.3 Sagittal, midsagittal, frontal or coronal, and transverse body planes.

It is essential for students to know the basic anatomical planes!

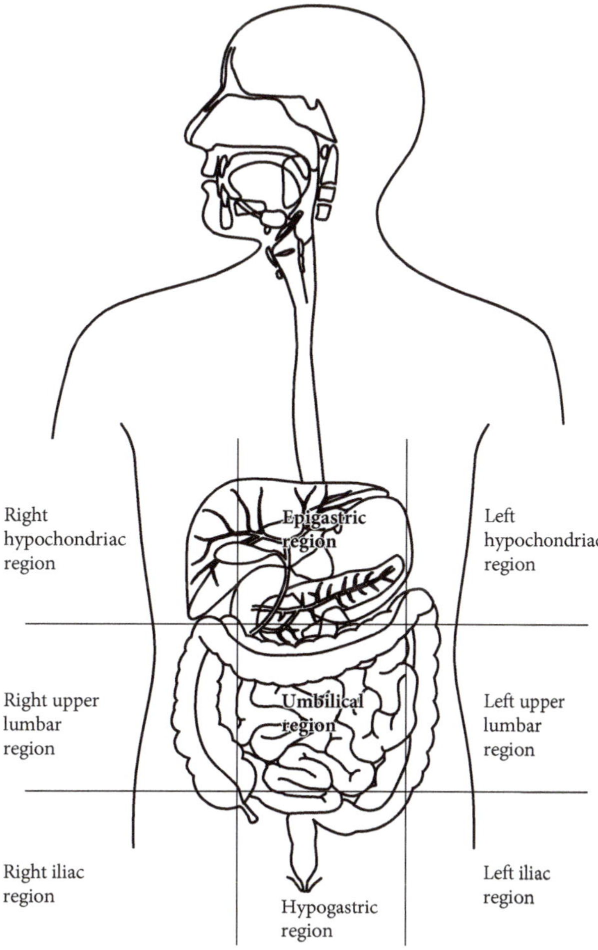

FIGURE 1.4 Color each of the nine abdominal surface areas a different color. NOTICE the organs located in each of the areas while you color.

Learn these abdominal areas and the organs that lie deep to each area!

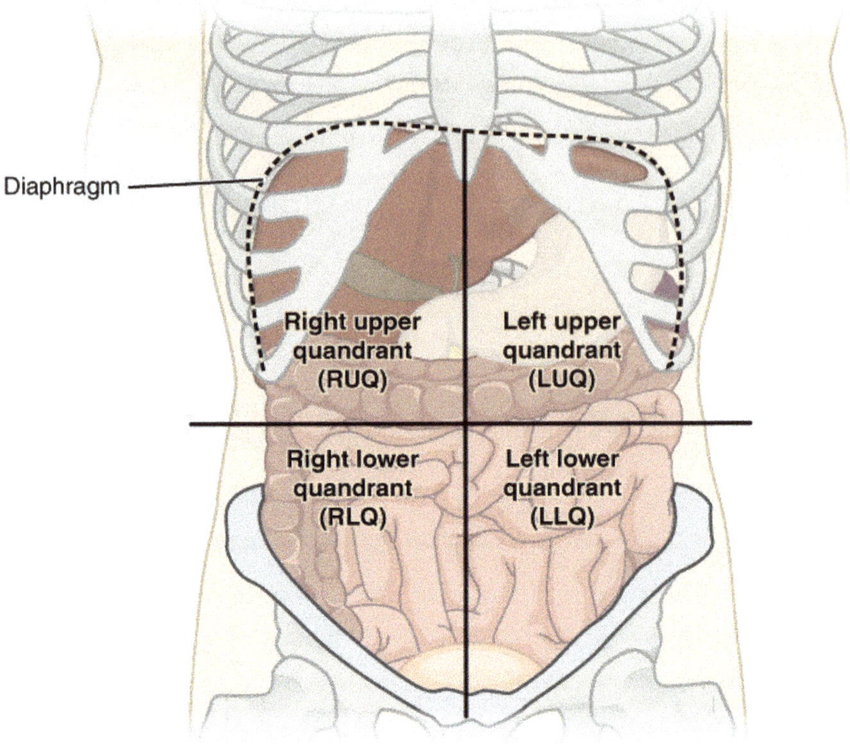

FIGURE 1.5 These four abdominal surface quadrants are used a great deal in clinical health care.

Clinically significant abdominal quadrants.

Lab Team Worksheet

LAB 1—BUILDING THE STUDENT TEAM

Name: **Date:**

Team Members present for Lab:

1.

2.

3.

4.

Collaborating as a Team, answer the following questions. Each Team will turn in *one* Lab Team Worksheet at the completion of Lab.

1. The ______________________________ is the standard reference position used in A&P and health care.

2. Physiology is the study of human ______________________________.

3. The basic ***concept*** of A&P is easily expressed as three letters: ______________________________.

4. Human organs are ________________ the way they are because of what they ________________.

5. The elbow is ________________ to the shoulder, but the shoulder is ________________ to the elbow.

6. A closed body cavity is ______________________________ to the environment outside the body.

7. Open body cavities are lined by ______________________________ membranes.

8. Mucous membranes provide ______________________________ immunity for the body.

Figure Credits

Fig. 1.1: Copyright © by OpenStax College (CC by 3.0) at https://commons.wikimedia.org/wiki/File:Opposition_CMX.jpg.

Fig. 1.2a: Copyright © by OpenStax College (CC by 3.0) at https://commons.wikimedia.org/wiki/File:Body_Cavities_Frontal_view.jpg.

Fig. 1.2b: Copyright © by OpenStax College (CC by 3.0) at https://commons.wikimedia.org/wiki/File:Body_Cavities_Lateral_view.jpg.

Fig. 1.3: Copyright © by David Richfield (CC BY-SA 4.0) at https://commons.wikimedia.org/wiki/File:Human_anatomy_planes.jpg.

Fig. 1.4: Adapted from: https://commons.wikimedia.org/wiki/File:Digestive_system_diagram_en.svg.

Fig. 1.5: Copyright © by Open Stax (CC by 3.0) at https://commons.wikimedia.org/wiki/File:Abdominal_Quadrants_English.jpg.

LAB 2

Chemistry Basics

Purpose of Lab and Desired Outcomes

1. Chemistry necessary to understanding human physiology
2. Atomic structure
3. Atomic elements—major and minor essential in physiology
4. Chemical bonding
5. Water and surface tension
6. Acidity and pH scale
7. Biological macromolecules
8. Enzymes
9. Oxidation/reduction reactions (redox)

Pre-Lab Worksheet

LAB 2—BASIC CHEMISTRY

Name: **Date:**

Each student should answer the following questions *before* coming to Lab.

In your own words, **DEFINE the following terms**. ***Do not*** just copy and paste answers! ALL of these questions can be defined or explained in a few words. Be ***concise*** when writing your answer.

1. Define chemistry.

____

____

____

2. List the six major chemical elements essential in human physiology.

____

____

____

3. What are the three types of chemical bonds? List them from the strongest to the weakest.

____

____

____

4. List four functions of water in the human body.

____

____

____

5. What does the pH scale measure?

______

______

______

6. List the four biochemicals that make up the human body.

______

______

______

7. What is an enzyme, and why are enzymes important in human physiology?

______

______

______

8. What is a redox reaction?

______

______

______

In-Lab Activities

1. Collection of student Pre-Lab Worksheets.
2. Instructor calls for QCs (Student Questions, Concerns, Confusions, and need for Clarification).
3. Brief instructor explanation of In-Lab Activities and desired outcomes from Lab time.
4. Follow the bullet points below to complete activities for the chemistry lab.
    - Utilizing a blank sheet of standard notebook paper, each Lab Team member will draw, to the best of their ability, a conceptual diagram of the hydrogen bonding that causes surface tension in water, or produce a graphic presentation (PPTs, Prezi, or Google Slides) in a virtual environment. Figure 5.5 in the *SS A&P*, 2nd Edition text will be helpful.
    - Collaborate with each other while doing your individual drawings. Utilize the *SS A&P* text. Look stuff up online. *Help* each other. *Ask* each other questions. *Teach* each other.
    - *Be creative!* Make your drawing graphic, colorful, and visual.
    - Individual student drawings will be turned in to the instructor/TA for evaluation, either in hard copy or digitally as a smartphone picture sent to the appropriate email.
    - Then, each Lab Team will collaborate to draw a conceptual diagram of the pH scale or produce a graphic presentation (PPTs, Prezi, or Google Slides) in a virtual environment.
5. A randomly selected Lab Team (roll of the dice) will discuss the Team graphics with the entire class.
    - Teams will be prepared to do Q&A with students and instructor.
    - Teams will take a picture of their graphics and electronically submit to instructor/TA.
    - Each Team will turn in one Team Worksheet to instructor/TA.
6. Instructor will complete "Major Takeaways" with the class.

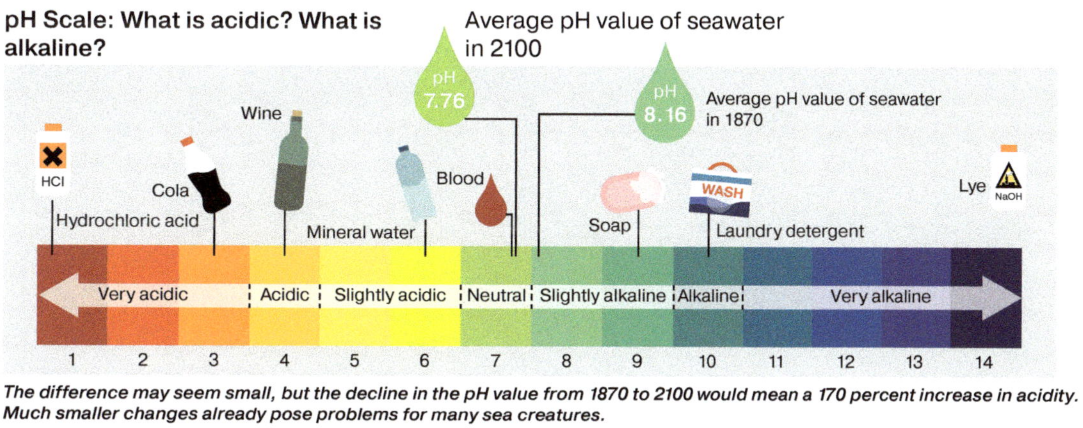

FIGURE 2.1 pH scale with examples.

Lab Team Worksheet

LAB 2—CHEMISTRY BASICS

Team Name: **Date:**

Team Members present for Lab:

1.

2.

3.

4.

Collaborating as a Team, answer the following questions. Each Team will turn in *one* Lab Team Worksheet at the completion of Lab.

1. A solution is a clear mixture of a ____________________ dissolved in a ____________________.

2. The body's "solvent" is ________________________________.

3. Hydrogen bonds between water molecules cause _________________________.

4. The two types of covalent bonds are ____________________ and ____________________.

5. The strongest chemical bond is the ______________________________ bond.

6. Water has a pH of ________________________________.

7. Acidity is caused by the concentration of _________________ ions or free _________________.

Figure Credit

Fig. 2.1: Copyright © by Heinrich-Boll-Stiftung (CC BY-SA 2.0) at https://commons.wikimedia.org/wiki/File:PH_Scale-_Acidic_vs._Basic_(Alkaline).png.

LAB 3

Cellular Energy Production

Purpose of Lab and Desired Outcomes

Participate in Individual and Lab Team Activities to gain insight and understanding into the following topics:

1. Cellular respiration—four phases
2. Endergonic and exergonic reactions
3. Catabolic and anabolic reactions
4. Aerobic and anaerobic reactions
5. Cellular energy storage—ATP
6. Redox reactions
7. Oxidative phosphorylation
8. Stargate molecule
9. The three primary sources of nutrition

Pre-Lab Worksheet

LAB 3—CELLULAR RESPIRATION

Name: **Date:**

Each individual student should answer the following questions *before* coming to Lab.

In your own words*, DEFINE the following terms. *Do not just copy and paste answers! ALL of these terms can be defined in a few words. Be ***concise*** when writing your answer.

1. Exergonic reaction ______________________________

2. Endergonic reaction ______________________________

3. Anabolic reaction ______________________________

4. Catabolic reaction ______________________________

5. Cellular respiration ______________________________

6. Aerobic reaction ______________________________

7. Anaerobic respiration ______________________________

8. ATP ______________________________

9. Redox reaction ______________________________

10. Oxidative phosphorylation ______________________________

In-Lab Activities

1. Collection of student Pre-Lab Worksheets.
2. Instructor calls for QCs (Student Questions, Concerns, Confusions, and need for Clarification).
3. Instructor explanation of In-Lab Activities and desired outcomes from Lab time.
4. Follow the bullet points below to gain insight into cellular respiration.
   - Utilizing a blank sheet of standard notebook paper, every student will draw, to the best of their ability, a conceptual diagram of cellular respiration or produce a graphic presentation (PPTs, Prezi, or Google Slides) in a virtual environment.
   - Collaborate with each other while doing your individual drawings. Look stuff up online. *Help* each other. *Ask* each other questions. *Teach* each other.
   - Individual student drawings will be turned in to the instructor/TA for evaluation.
   - Each Team will then draw a conceptual diagram of cellular respiration on a large sheet of paper or produce a graphic presentation (PPTs, Prezi, or Google Slides) in a virtual environment.
5. A randomly selected Lab Team (roll of the dice) will discuss their graphic with the entire class by sticking/hanging their graphic and leading a discussion about it.
   - Teams will be prepared to do Q&A with students and instructor.
   - Teams will take a picture of their graphic and electronically submit it to instructor/TA.
   - Each Team will turn in one Team Worksheet to instructor/TA.
6. Instructor will complete "Major Takeaways" with the class.

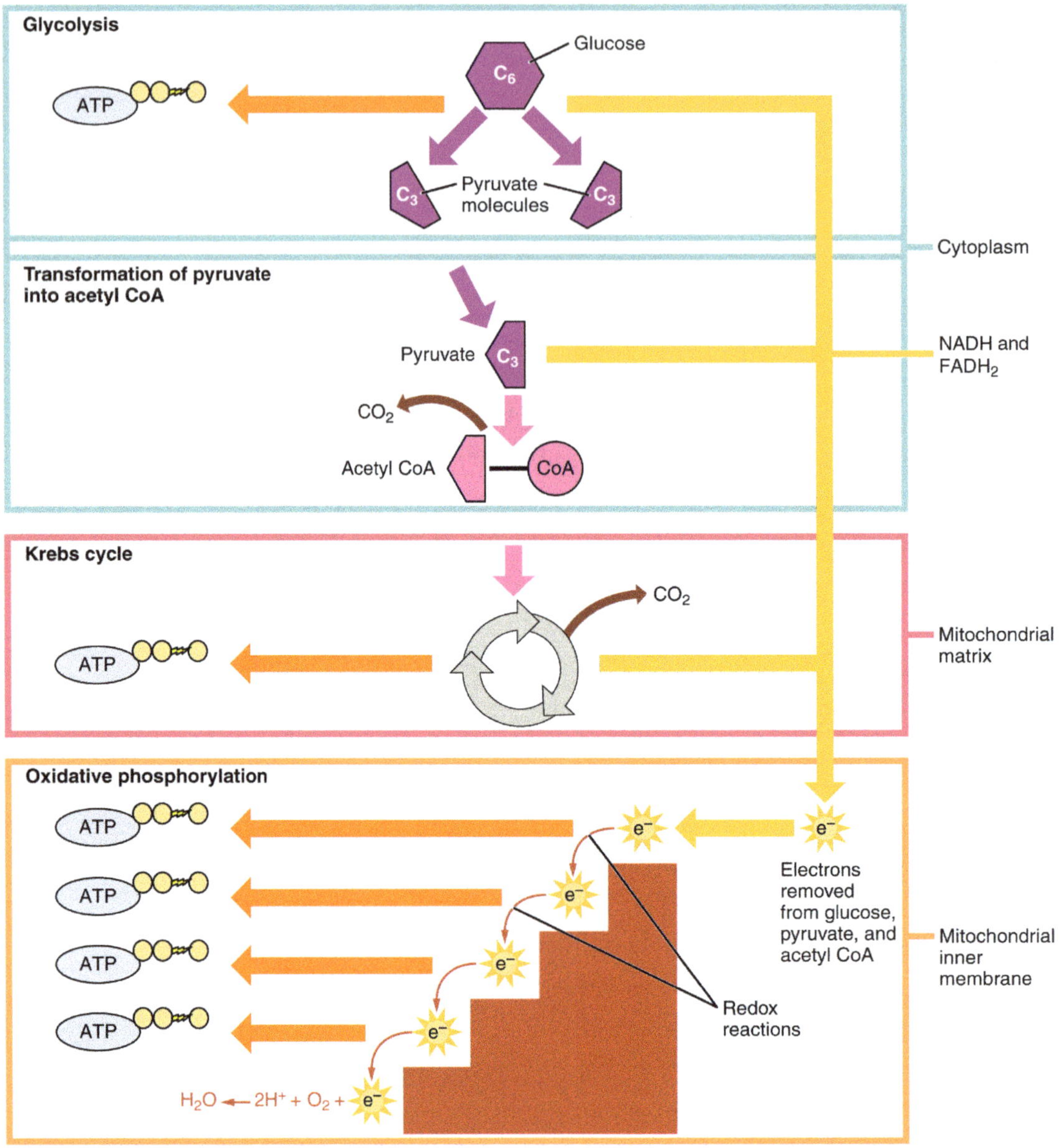

FIGURE 3.1 Excellent simplistic summary of cellular respiration.

Simplistic conceptual diagram demonstrating the essence of cellular respiration.

Lab Team Worksheet

LAB 3—CELLULAR RESPIRATION

Team Name: **Date:**

Team Members present for Lab:

1.

2.

3.

4.

Collaborating as a Team, answer the following questions. Each Team will turn in *one* Lab Team Worksheet at the completion of Lab.

1. Two types of cell transport occur in the ETC: facilitated diffusion and active transport.

    a. What is actively transported? ____________________

    b. What was the energy source for this active transport? ____________________

    c. Where did facilitated diffusion occur? ____________________

2. In oxidation, a molecule ____________________ electrons, whereas in reduction, a molecule will ____________________ electrons.

3. Glycolysis produces two molecules of ____________________

4. ____________________ is the "stargate" molecule leading from the bridge into the Krebs or citric acid cycle.

5. A portal that leads into another level or realm is called a ____________________ .

6. List the two molecules (B vitamins) that carry high-energy electrons from glycolysis, the bridge, and the citric cycle into the ETC.

____

____

7. Most energy (ATP) is produced by the ETC. Since the first three stages of CR do not produce large amounts of ATP, what do those first three phases produce that is essential for the ETC to function?

____

Figure Credit

Fig. 3.1: Copyright © by OpenStax College (CC by 3.0) at https://commons.wikimedia.org/wiki/File:2503_Cellular_Respiration.jpg.

LAB 4

Protein Synthesis

Purpose of Lab and Desired Outcomes

Participate in Individual and Lab Team Activities to gain insight and understanding into the following topics:

1. Protein synthesis
2. DNA and RNA
3. Transcription and translation
4. Ribosomes
5. Golgi apparatus
6. Vesicles
7. Exocytosis
8. Protein structure and importance

Pre-Lab Worksheet

LAB 4—PROTEIN SYNTHESIS

Name: **Date:**

Before coming to Lab, each student should complete the reading assignment for this Lab activity, then answer the following questions:

1. Protein synthesis produces ______________________.

2. The cell's "protein factory" is the ______________________.

3. Conceptually, __________________ is the source of the "recipe" for each individual protein.

4. Transcription takes place in the ______________________.

5. Translation takes place in the ______________________.

6. The genetic code for protein structure is contained in ______________________.

7. List four examples of proteins that are essential to human function.

____

____

____

In-Lab Activities

1. Collection of student Pre-Lab Worksheets.
2. Instructor calls for QCs (Student Questions, Concerns, Confusions, and need for clarification).
3. Instructor explanation of In-Lab Activities and desired outcomes from Lab time.
4. Follow the bullet points below to gain insight into protein synthesis.
   - Utilizing a blank sheet of standard notebook paper, each student will draw, to the best of their ability, a conceptual diagram of protein synthesis or produce a graphic presentation (PPTs, Prezi, or Google Slides) in a virtual environment.
   - Collaborate with each other while doing your individual drawings. Look stuff up online. *Help* each other. *Ask* each other questions. *Teach* each other.
   - Individual student drawings will be turned in to the instructor/TA for evaluation.
   - Each Team will then draw a conceptual diagram of protein synthesis on a large sheet of paper or produce a graphic presentation (PPTs, Prezi, or Google Slides) in a virtual environment.
5. A randomly (roll of the dice) selected Lab Team will discuss their graphics with the entire class by leading a class discussion of their graphic.
   - Teams will be prepared to do Q&A with students and instructor.
   - All Teams will take a picture of their graphic and electronically submit it to instructor/TA for review.
   - Each Team will turn in one Team Worksheet to instructor/TA.
6. Instructor will complete "Major Takeaways" with the class.

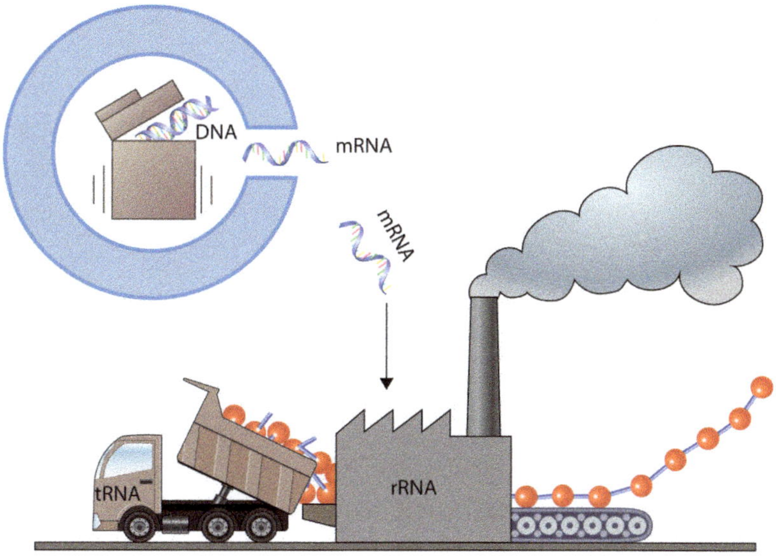

FIGURE 4.1 Simplistic summary of protein synthesis.

Simplistic conceptual graphic showing the essential aspects of protein synthesis.

Lab Team Worksheet

LAB 4—PROTEIN SYNTHESIS

Team Name: **Date:**

Team Members present for Lab:

1.

2.

3.

4.

Collaborating as a Team, answer the following questions. Each Team will turn in *one* Lab Team Worksheet at the completion of Lab.

1. What are the two primary steps in the process of protein synthesis?

____

____

2. The ______________________ is referred to as the cell's "protein factory."

3. Protein synthesis produces ______________________.

4. Translation takes place in the ______________________.

5. Transcription takes place in the ______________________.

6. ______________________ are the basic "building blocks" of proteins.

7. The protein that lowers blood glucose is ______________________.

8. List two conceptual examples demonstrating the importance of proteins in human physiology.

____

____

Figure Credit

Fig. 4.1: Julissa Alveres, Super Simple Anatomy and Physiology: The Ultimate Learning Tool, ed. Nelson Kraus, p. 205. Copyright © 2017 by Cognella, Inc. Reprinted with permission.

LAB 5

Concepts of Cellular Biology

Purpose of Lab and Desired Outcomes

Participate in Individual and Lab Team Activities to gain insight and understanding into the following topics:

1. Basic cell biology
2. Structure of a typical human cell
3. Cell membrane—structure and importance
4. Major intracellular organelles
5. Plasma membrane extensions or modifications
6. Functions of mitosis
7. Basic concept of anatomy and physiology

Pre-Lab Worksheet

LAB 5—CONCEPTS OF CELLULAR BIOLOGY

Name: **Date:**

Before coming to Lab, each student should complete the reading assignment for this Lab activity, then answer the following questions:

1. The structural unit of the human body is the ______________________________.

2. The functional unit of the human body is the ______________________________.

3. List the three parts of the human cell from outside the cell to inside.

   ____

   ____

   ____

4. The cell membrane is ____________, allowing some substances to pass while blocking other substances.

5. Some cells have extensions of the cell membrane that allow them to perform specific functions. List the three cell membrane extensions or modifications.

   ____

   ____

   ____

6. The SPPLBL is about 20 percent ____________________________ , providing stability to the cell membrane.

In-Lab Activities

1. Collection of student Pre-Lab Worksheets.
2. Instructor calls for QCs (Student Questions, Concerns, Confusions, and need for Clarification).
3. Instructor explanation of In-Lab Activities and desired outcomes from Lab time.
4. Lab Teams will draw a composite human cell as shown in Figure 7.1 in the 2nd edition of *SS A&P* text on a large piece of paper or produce a graphic presentation (PPTs, Prezi, or Google Slides) in a virtual environment.
5. In addition, Lab Teams will draw a cell membrane (SPPLBL—Semipermeable Phospho-Lipid Bilayer) as seen in Figure 7.2 in the 2nd edition of *SS A&P* text on a large piece of paper or produce a graphic presentation (PPTs, Prezi, or Google Slides) in a virtual environment.

   While working on the graphics in #4 and #5 above, Teams are encouraged to:
   - Discuss the graphic among Team members.
   - Ask each other questions.
   - Teach each other.
   - Prepare verbal explanations of the graphics.
   - Be prepared to share the graphics and explanations with the entire lab.
   - Complete the Team Lab Worksheet and turn it in at the end of Lab.
6. Randomly selected Lab Teams (roll of the dice) will discuss their cell and cell membrane graphics with the entire class.
   - Teams will be prepared to do Q&A discussion with students and instructor.
   - Each Team will take a picture of their final cell and SPPLBL graphics and electronically submit it to instructor/TA.
   - Each Team will turn in one Team Worksheet to instructor/TA.
7. Instructor will complete “Major Takeaways” with the class.

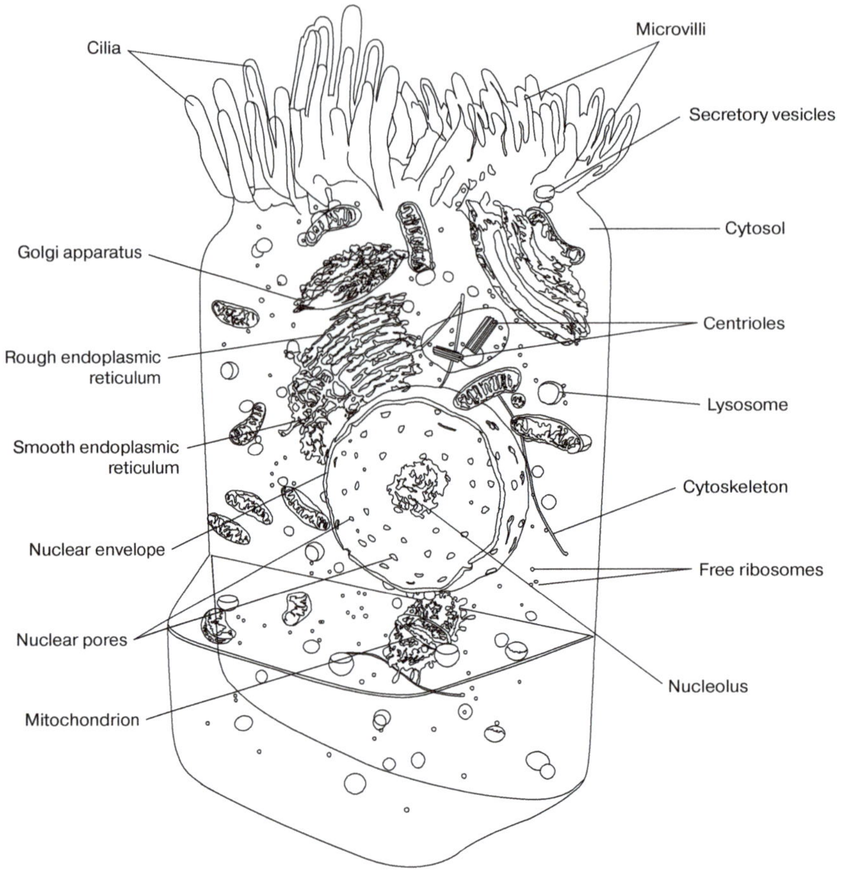

FIGURE 5.1 Color in each part of this composite cell, and write out the function of that structure.

The cell membrane is the key to movement of substances into and out of the cell.

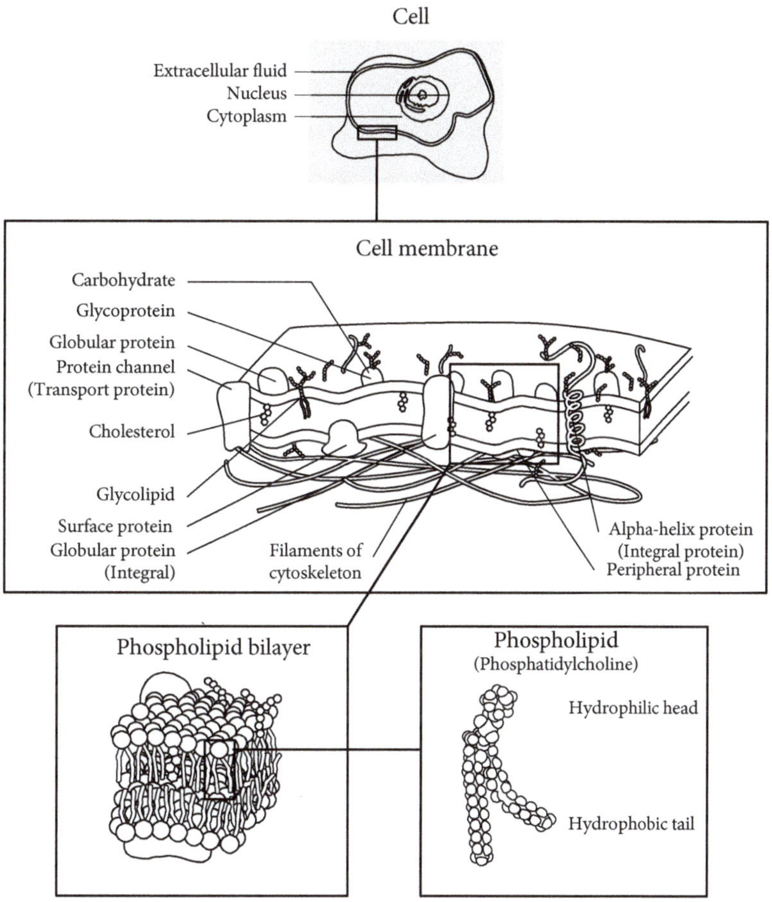

FIGURE 5.2 Sequential demonstration of the cell down to molecular structure.

Make sure you understand all the components of the cell membrane, down to the molecular level.

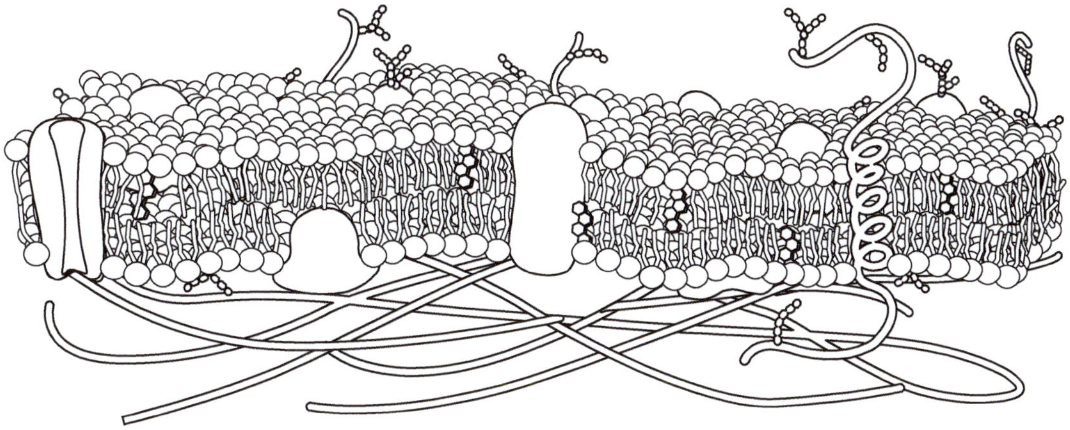

FIGURE 5.3 Color this conceptual diagram of an SPPLBL, and label the structures you color.

Opportunity to review by labeling structures of the cell membrane.

Lab Team Worksheet

LAB 5—CONCEPTS OF CELLULAR BIOLOGY

Team Name: **Date:**

Team Members present for Lab:

1.

2.

3.

4.

Collaborating as a Team, answer the following questions. Each Team will turn in *one* Lab Team Worksheet at the completion of Lab.

1. Anatomy is the study of human ______________________________.

2. Physiology is the study of human ______________________________.

3. The basic *concept* of A&P is easily expressed as three letters: ______________________________.

4. Human organs are ________________ the way they are because of what they ________________.

5. Mitosis provides two functions to the body. What are they?

   ____

   ____

6. The Golgi apparatus ______________ and ______________proteins produced by the rough ER and free cytoplasmic ribosomes.

7. What is the six-letter abbreviation that describes the plasma membrane? ____________________

Figure Credits

Fig. 5.1: Copyright © by Blausen.com staff (CC by 3.0) at https://commons.wikimedia.org/wiki/File:Blausen_0208_CellAnatomy.png.

Fig. 5.2: Copyright © by Dhatfield (CC BY-SA 3.0) at https://commons.wikimedia.org/wiki/File:Cell_membrane_detailed_diagram_4.svg.

Fig. 5.3: Source: https://commons.wikimedia.org/wiki/File:Cell_membrane_detailed_diagram_blank.svg.

LAB 6

Membrane Transport

Purpose of Lab and Desired Outcomes

Participate in Individual and Lab Team Activities to gain insight and understanding into the following topics:

1. Cell membrane structure
2. Diffusion—simple and facilitated
3. Osmosis
4. Tonicity

Pre-Lab Worksheet

LAB 6—CONCEPTS OF CELLULAR BIOLOGY

Name: **Date:**

Each student should answer the following questions *before* coming to Lab.
Complete reading assignments (chapter 7 in *SS A&P* text, 2nd Edition) for this Lab Activity. Then answer the following questions:

1. The structural unit of the human body is the ______________________________.

2. The functional unit of the human body is the ______________________________.

3. List the three parts of the human cell from outside the cell to inside the cell.

   ____

   ____

   ____

4. The cell membrane is ________________________, allowing some substances to pass while blocking other substances.

5. The random movement of molecules from higher to lower concentration is called ______________.

6. Name the two types of diffusion.

   ____

   ____

7. The ability of a solution to change the volume or tone of a cell through osmosis is called

   ______________________________.

In-Lab Activities

1. Collection of student Pre-Lab Worksheets.
2. Instructor calls for QCs (Student Questions, Concerns, Confusions, and need for Clarification).
3. Instructor explanation of In-Lab Activities and desired outcomes from Lab time.
4. On a large sheet of paper, Lab Teams will draw a graphic demonstrating the concept of simple and facilitated diffusion. Or produce a graphic presentation (PPTs, Prezi, or Google Slides) of diffusion when in a virtual environment.
5. On a second large sheet of paper, Lab Teams will draw a graphic demonstrating the concepts of tonicity. Or produce a graphic presentation (PPTs, Prezi, or Google Slides) of tonicity when in a virtual environment.

While working on the graphics in #4 and #5 above, Teams are encouraged to:

- Discuss the graphic among Team members.
- Ask each other questions.
- Teach each other.
- Prepare verbal explanations of the graphics.
- Be prepared to share the graphics and explanations with the entire lab.
- Complete the Team Lab Worksheet and turn it in at the end of Lab.

6. Randomly selected Lab Teams (roll of the dice) will discuss their graphics with the entire class.
   - Teams will be prepared to do Q&A ***discussion*** with students and instructor.
   - Each Team will take a picture of their graphics and electronically submit it to instructor/TA.
   - Each Team will turn in one Team Worksheet to instructor/TA.
7. Instructor will complete "Major Takeaways" with the class.

Lab Team Worksheet

LAB 6—MEMBRANE TRANSPORT

Team Name: **Date:**

Team Members present for Lab:

1.

2.

3.

4.

Collaborating as a Team, answer the following questions. Each Team will turn in *one* Lab Team Worksheet at the completion of Lab.

1. The movement of water through a semipermeable membrane toward a solute concentration is called

   ______________________.

2. What are the three things required for osmosis to occur?

   ____

   ____

   ____

3. Figuratively, osmotically active solutes "______________________."

4. Simple diffusion is a ______________________ process and does not require the presence of

   ______________________.

5. A human RBC placed in a hypertonic solution of salt would ______________________.

6. A human RBC placed in a hypertonic solution of sugar would ______________________.

7. A human RBC placed in an isotonic solution of salt or sugar would ______________________.

LAB 7

Tissue Identification

Purpose of Lab and Desired Outcomes

Participate in Individual and Lab Team Activities to gain insight and understanding into the following topics:

1. Nine specific types of epithelial tissue
2. Thirteen types of connective tissue
3. Three types of muscle tissue
4. Nervous tissue
5. Conceptual function of each of the four primary types of tissue

Pre-Lab Worksheet

LAB 7—TISSUE IDENTIFICATION

Name: **Date:**

Before coming to Lab, each student should complete the reading assignment for this Lab activity, then answer the following questions:

1. List the four primary types of tissue in the human body.

____

____

____

____

2. Epithelial tissue is named based on the number of ______________________________ and the ______________________________ of cells at the apical surface.

3. Simple cuboidal epithelium has apical cells shaped like little ______________________________.

4. List the three general types of connective tissue.

____

____

____

In-Lab Activities

1. Collection of student Pre-Lab Worksheets.
2. Instructor calls for QCs (Student Questions, Concerns, Confusions, and need for Clarification).
3. Instructor explanation of In-Lab Activities and desired outcomes from Lab time.
4. Teams will locate an online site or multiple sites showing histological examples of tissue. Choose one or more sites to utilize in the following activity.
   - Discuss characteristics of the four primary tissues based on reading *SS A&P* as well as other A&P or histology references.
   - Utilizing six large sheets of paper, teams will draw a cross dividing each page into four equal squares, like windowpanes.
   - Draw graphic representations of a total of twenty-four different types of tissue discussed in the 2nd Edition of the *SS A&P* text. Or produce a graphic presentation (PPTs, Prezi, or Google Slides) of the tissues in a virtual environment.
     - eight of the nine types of epithelial tissue
     - twelve of the thirteen types of connective tissue
     - all three types of muscle tissue
     - nervous tissue showing a classic multipolar neuron
5. While working on the graphics to complete #4 above, Teams are encouraged to:
   - Discuss the graphics among Team members.
   - Ask each other questions.
   - Teach each other.
   - Prepare verbal explanations of the graphics.
   - Be prepared to share the graphics and explanations with the entire Lab.
   - Complete the Team Lab Worksheet for turn-in at the end of Lab.
6. Randomly selected (throw of the dice) Lab Teams lead a class discussion about the specific tissue types.
   - Teams will be prepared to do Q&A with students and instructor.
   - All Teams will take a picture (on a smartphone) of their graphics and electronically submit it to instructor/TA.
   - Each Team will turn in one Team Worksheet to instructor/TA.
7. Instructor will complete "Major Takeaways" with the class.

Lab Team Worksheet

LAB 7—TISSUE IDENTIFICATION

Team Name: **Date:**

Team Members present for Lab:

1.

2.

3.

4.

Collaborating as a Team, answer the following questions. Each Team will turn in *one* Lab Team Worksheet at the completion of Lab.

1. Skeletal muscle is also called ______________________ or ______________________.
2. Visceral muscle is also called ______________________ or ______________________.
3. Cells in connective tissue are suspended in a ______________________.
4. ______________________ is the most common type of cartilage.
5. An identifying characteristic of cardiac muscle is ______________________ discs.
6. Visceral muscle is ________________ the way it is because of what it ________________.
7. The cells at the apical surface of transitional epithelium are called ________________ cells.

LAB 8

Histology and Tissue Organization

Purpose of Lab and Desired Outcomes

Participate in Individual and Lab Team Activities to gain insight and understanding into the following topics:

1. Histology
2. Primary types of tissue
3. Naming of epithelium
4. Types of connective tissue
5. Types of muscle tissue
6. Nervous tissue

Pre-Lab Worksheet

LAB 8—HISTOLOGY AND TISSUE ORGANIZATION

Name: **Date:**

Before coming to Lab, each student should complete the reading assignment for this Lab activity, then answer the following questions:

1. Histology is the ______________________ of ______________________.

2. The tissues are ______________________ the way they are because of what they ______________________.

3. Epithelium ______________________ and ______________________.

4. Epithelial tissues are named based on two characteristics. Name them.

   ____

   ____

5. All epithelium has a free or ______________________ surface.

6. Conceptually, muscle creates ______________________ in the body.

In-Lab Activities

1. Collection of student Pre-Lab Worksheets.
2. Instructor calls for QCs (Student Questions, Concerns, Confusions, and need for Clarification).
3. Instructor explanation of In-Lab Activities and desired outcomes from Lab time.
4. Lab teams will draw a cross dividing a large sheet of paper into four equal squares, like windowpanes. Or teams will produce a graphic presentation (PPTs, Prezi, or Google Slides) in a virtual environment. Team will draw an example of each of the four primary types of tissue (E, C, M, N), one per "pane."
    - Indicate *graphically* (in pictures, not words) what each of those tissue types does. Refer to the H_2O Sheet in chapter 2 of *SS A&P* text, 2nd Edition.
5. On a separate large sheet of paper, Lab Teams will draw a graphic (picture) demonstrating how the four tissues combine in an organ. Teams can choose any organ they wish to draw. Or teams will produce a graphic presentation (PPTs, Prezi, or Google Slides) in a virtual environment. While working on the graphics in #4 and #5, Teams are encouraged to:
    - Discuss the graphics among Team members.
    - Ask each other questions.
    - Teach each other.
    - Prepare verbal explanations of the graphics.
    - Be prepared to share the graphics and explanations with the entire lab.
    - Complete the Team Lab Worksheet for turn-in at the end of Lab.
6. Randomly selected Lab Teams (roll of the dice) will lead a *class discussion* (more than just a presentation of the graphic) by asking colleagues questions about the graphic.
    - Teams will be prepared to do Q&A with students and instructor.
    - Each Team will take a picture (with a smartphone) of their graphics and electronically submit it to instructor/TA.
    - Each Team will turn in one Team Worksheet to instructor/TA.
    - Each Team will recycle the pages.
7. Instructor will complete "Major Takeaways" with the class.

Cells	Location	Function
Simple squamous epithelium 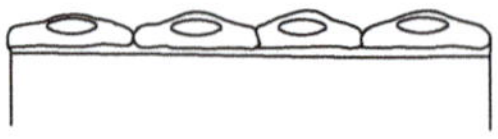	Air sacs of lungs and the lining of the heart, blood vessels, and lymphatic vessels	Allows materials to pass through by diffusion and filtration, and secretes lubricating substance
Simple cuboidal epithelium 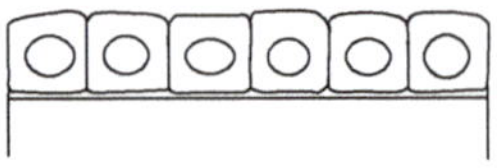	In ducts and secretory portions of small glands and in kidney tubules	Secretes and absorbs
Simple columnar epithelium 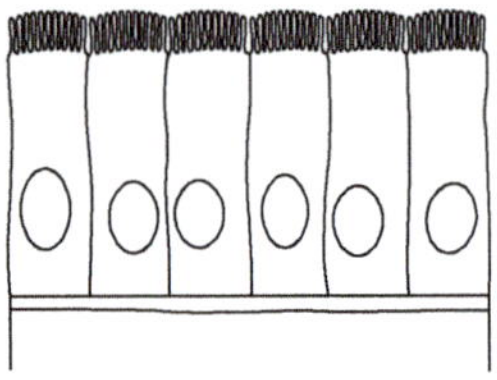	Ciliated tissues are in bronchi, uterine tubes, and uterus; smooth (nonciliated tissues) are in the digestive tract, bladder	Absorbs; it also secretes mucous and enzymes
Pseudostratified columnar epithelium 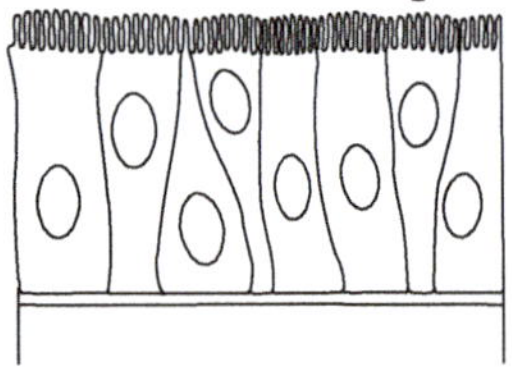	Ciliated tissue lines the trachea and much of the upper respiratory tract	Secretes mucus; ciliated tissue moves mucus
Stratified squamous epithelium 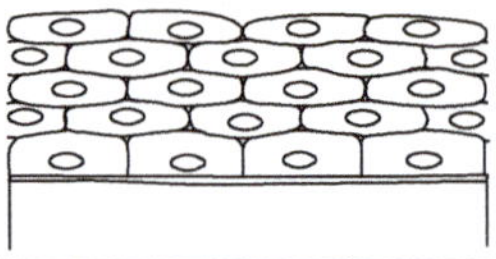	Lines the esophagus, mouth, and vagina	Protects against abrasion
Stratified cuboidal epithelium 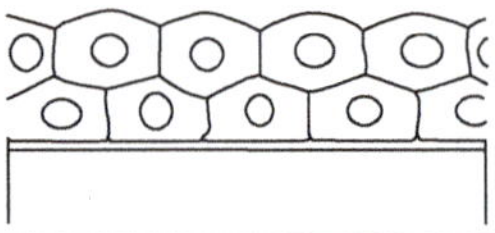	Sweat glands, salivary glands, and the mammary glands	Protective tissue
Stratified columnar epithelium 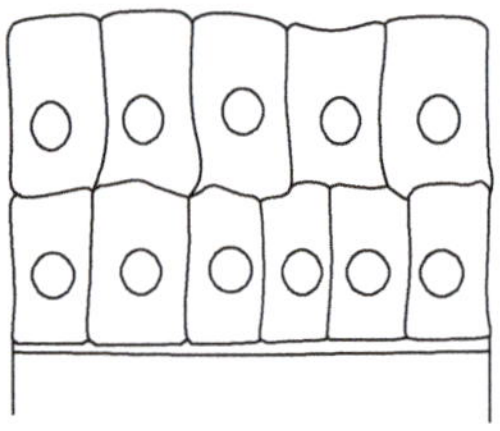	The male urethra and the ducts of some glands	Secretes and protects
Transitional epithelium 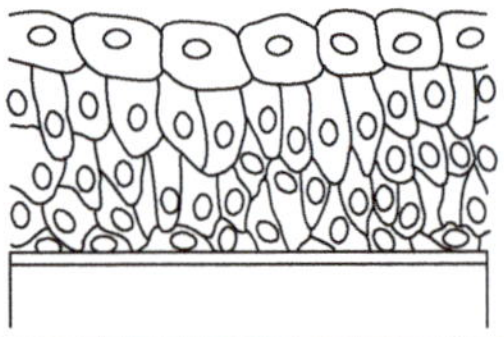	Lines the bladder, uretha, and the ureters	Allows the urinary organs to expand and stretch

FIGURE 8.1 Coloring and review opportunity regarding epithelial tissue.

How are specific types of epithelial tissue named?

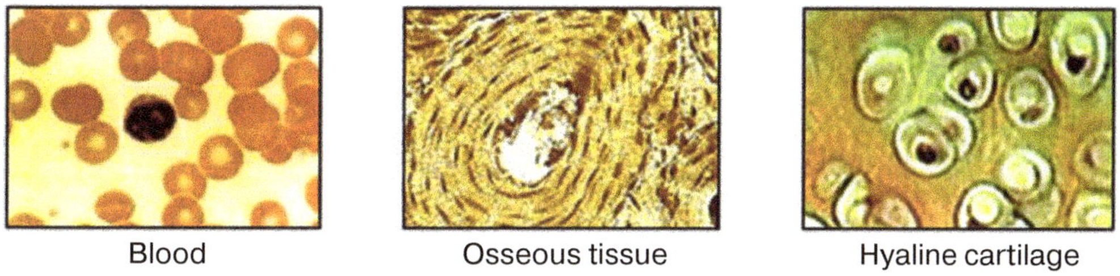

FIGURE 8.2 Three types of connective tissue. Name and describe at least nine specific types of connective tissue.

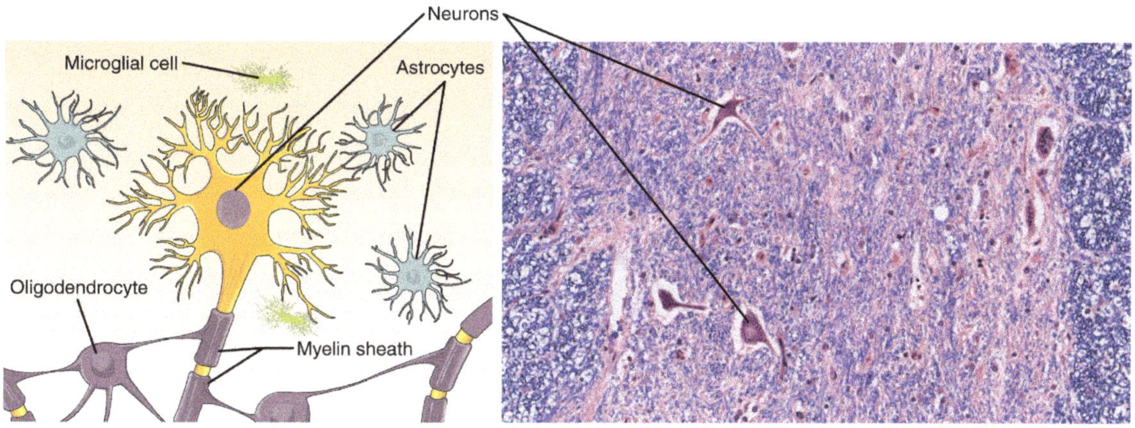

FIGURE 8.3 Nerve cells and glial support cells for review.

The neuron is the functional and structural unit of the nervous system, supported by neuroglial cells.

Lab Team Worksheet

LAB 8—HISTOLOGY AND TISSUE ORGANIZATION

Team Name: **Date:**

Team Members present for Lab:

1.

2.

3.

4.

Collaborating as a Team, answer the following questions. Each Team will turn in *one* Lab Team Worksheet at the completion of Lab.

1. Conceptually, nervous tissue provides ______________________ in the body.

2. The matrix in blood is the ______________________.

3. All connective tissue contains a ______________________.

4. Skeletal muscle is also called ____________________ or ____________________.

5. Visceral muscle is also called ____________________ or ____________________.

6. ____________________ and ____________________ are both fluid connective tissues.

7. The most common type of cartilage is ______________________.

Figure Credits

Fig. 8.1: Copyright © by OpenStax College (CC by 3.0) at https://commons.wikimedia.org/wiki/File:423_Table_04_02_Summary_of_Epithelial_Tissue_CellsN.jpg.

Fig. 8.2: Source: https://commons.wikimedia.org/wiki/File:Illu_connective_tissues_2.jpg.

Fig. 8.3: Copyright © by OpenStax College (CC by 3.0) at https://commons.wikimedia.org/wiki/File:416_Nervous_Tissue-new.jpg.

LAB 9

Integumentary System (Skin)

Purpose of Lab and Desired Outcomes

Participate in Individual and Lab Team Activities to gain insight and understanding into the following topics:

1. Skin
2. Skin layers
3. Epidermis
4. Dermis
5. Subcutaneous layer
6. Burns
7. Skin cancer

Pre-Lab Worksheet

LAB 9—INTEGUMENTARY SYSTEM

Name: **Date:**

Each student will answer the following questions *before* coming to Lab.

Complete the reading assignments for this Lab Activity. Then, answer the following questions:

1. Conceptually, the skin provides the following two basic functions:

   ____

   ____

2. The skin is ______________ the way it is because of what it ______________.

3. The ______________ is referred to as the "true" skin.

4. There are two different types of skin, depending on the location in the body. What are they?

   ____

   ____

5. All epithelium have a free ______________ surface.

6. List the two layers of the dermis (superficial first, deep second).

   ____

   ____

In-Lab Activities

1. Collection of student Pre-Lab Worksheets.
2. Instructor calls for QCs (Student Questions, Concerns, Confusions, and need for Clarification).
3. Instructor explanation of In-Lab Activities and desired outcomes from Lab time.
4. Lab Teams will draw on one side of a large piece of paper, the Skin Flow Chart, Figure 9.1 in the *SS A&P* text, 2nd Edition or produce a graphic presentation (PPTs, Prezi, or Google Slides) in a virtual environment.
5. On another large piece of paper, Lab Teams will draw a visual representation of a Cross Section of Human Skin, Figure 9.2 or produce a graphic presentation (PPTs, Prezi, or Google Slides) in a virtual environment.
    - While working on the graphics in #4 and #5, Teams are encouraged to:
        - Discuss the graphics using any models available.
        - Ask each other questions.
        - Teach each other.
        - Prepare verbal explanations of the graphics.
        - Be prepared to share the graphics and explanations with the entire Lab.
        - Complete the Team Lab Worksheet for turn-in at the end of Lab.
6. Randomly selected (roll of the dice) Lab Teams lead a class discussion about the graphic.
    - Teams will be prepared to do Q&A with students and instructor.
    - All Teams will take a picture (with a smartphone) of their graphics and electronically submit it to instructor/TA.
    - Each Team will turn in one Team Worksheet to instructor/TA.
7. Instructor will complete “Major Takeaways” with the class.

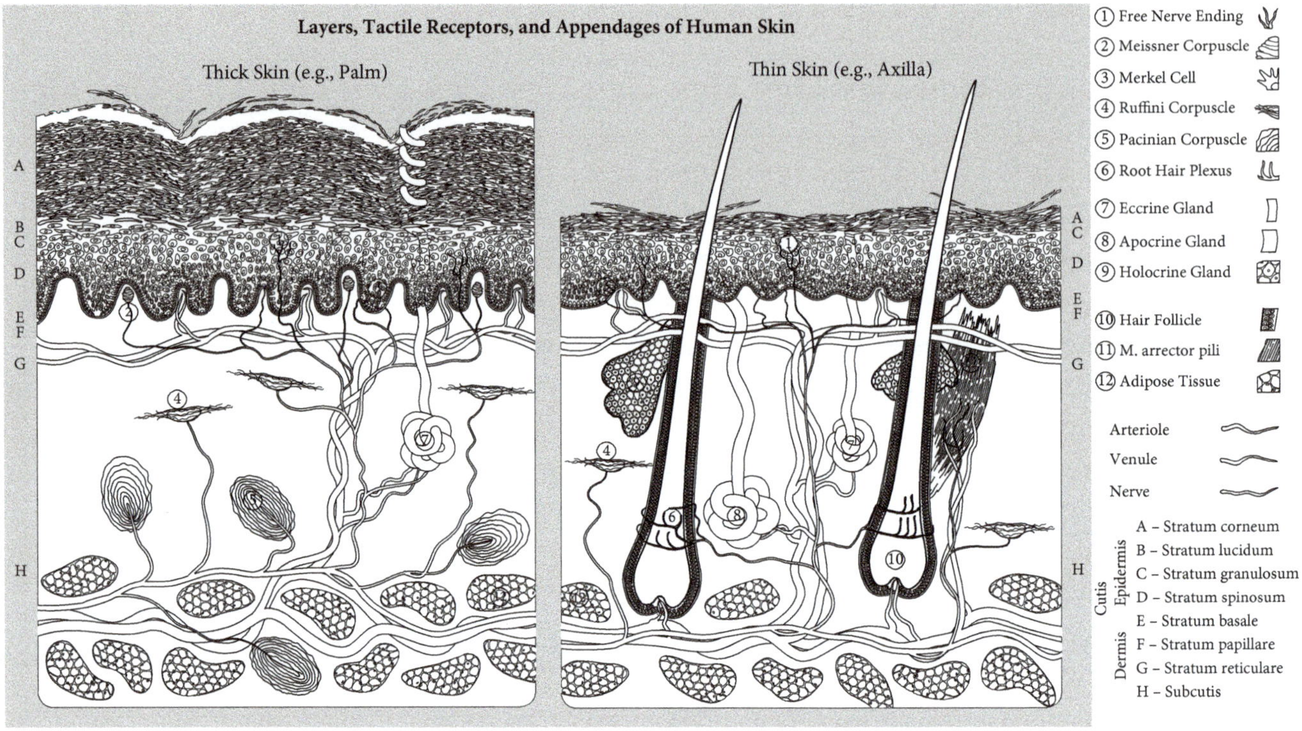

FIGURE 9.1 Color and review time with this cross-section of human skin.

Name the sensory receptors found in the skin.

Lab Team Worksheet

LAB 9—INTEGUMENTARY SYSTEM

Team Name: **Date:**

Team Members present for Lab:

1.

2.

3.

4.

Collaborating as a Team, answer the following questions. Each Team will turn in *one* Lab Team Worksheet at the completion of Lab.

1. What are the two conceptual functions of skin?

____

____

2. The dermis is called the ____________________ skin.

3. Thick skin is found in two areas of the body. Where are they?

____

____

4. Thick skin is ________________ the way it is because of what it ________________.

5. The most serious type of skin cancer is ____________________.

6. List the two types of sweat glands.

____

____

Figure Credit

Fig. 9.1: Copyright © by Guido4 (CC BY-SA 4.0) at https://commons.wikimedia.org/wiki/File:06_Hegasy_Skin_Layers_Receptors_Wiki_EN_CCBYSA.png.

LAB 10

Skeletal System—"Dem Bones"

Purpose of Lab and Desired Outcomes

Participate in Individual and Lab Team Activities to gain insight and understanding into the following topics:

1. Anatomy of a long bone
2. Classification of bones
3. Axial skeleton
4. Appendicular skeleton
5. Joints (particularly the knee)

Pre-Lab Worksheet

LAB 10—SKELETAL SYSTEM

Name: **Date:**

Complete the reading assignments for this Lab Activity. Then, answer the following questions:

1. The skeletal system provides ______________________ and ______________________.

2. ______________________ is the major organ of the skeletal system.

3. The bones of the skeleton are classified by their size and shape. What are the four classifications of bone?

____

____

____

____

4. Bones are ______________________ the way they are because of what they ______________________.

5. The axial skeleton is comprised of the skull, vertebral column, thoracic cage, and the ______________________ bone.

In-Lab Activities

1. Collection of student Pre-Lab Worksheets.
2. Instructor calls for QCs (Student Questions, Concerns, Confusions, and need for Clarification).
3. Instructor explanation of In-Lab Activities and desired outcomes from Lab time.
4. Utilizing anatomical models, an articulated skeleton, free bones, online resources, and pictures, student Teams will work collaboratively to identify the following bony structures:
   - Axial skeleton
     - Skull—including the mandible
       - Surface bones of the cranium
       - Major facial bones
       - Mandible—major aspects of mandible
       - Cranial fossa
   - Major openings of the skull
     - Canals—optic and hypoglossal
     - Foramina—oval, rotundum, etc.
     - Fissures—superior orbital
   - Identify what occupies or runs through the major openings
   - Vertebral column
     - Cervical
     - Thoracic
     - Sacral
     - Coccyx
   - Thoracic cage
     - Ribs
     - Sternum—three parts
   - Hyoid bone—uniqueness and forensic importance
   - Appendicular skeleton
     - Upper extremity
       - Pectoral girdle—clavicle and scapula
       - Upper extremity
         Humerus
         Ulna
         Radius
         Carpals—eight bones
         Hand—metacarpals and phalanges
     - Lower extremity
       - Pelvic girdle—four bones
         Sacrum—part of the axial skeleton
         Coccyx—part of the axial skeleton
         Left and right os coxae—pelvic bones—part of the appendicular skeleton
       - Femur
       - Tibia

        - Fibula
        - Tarsal bones
          Talus
          Calcaneus
        - Foot—metatarsals and phalanges
- Joints
    - TMJ—temporomandibular
    - Shoulder
    - Elbow
    - Hip—femur and pelvis
    - Knee—joint of emphasis!
        - Classic synovial joint
        - High clinical significance
        - Identify at least thirteen specific structures in the knee (see *SS A&P* text, 2nd Edition, page 125)
    - Ankle

While working to identify the above structures, Teams will concurrently do the following:

- On a large sheet of paper, Lab Teams will draw a cross dividing the page into four equal squares, like windowpanes.
- Draw an example of each of the four categories of bone classification:
    - Long
    - Short
    - Flat
    - Irregular
- Or produce a graphic presentation (PPTs, Prezi, or Google Slides) in a virtual environment.

On a separate sheet of paper, Teams will draw one of the bones (your choice) listed below (rib through tibia). Teams must indicate how to differentiate whether the bone is found on the left or right side of the body. Produce a graphic presentation (PPTs, Prezi, or Google Slides) in a virtual environment.

If there are more than six Teams, then the instructor will assign specific bones to each team.

- Rib
- Clavicle
- Scapula
- Humerus
- Femur
- Tibia

Teams must indicate on the above drawing exactly how to tell if the bone is left or right.

Teams will prepare to explain their graphic during class discussion time in #5.

5. Randomly selected Lab Teams will discuss graphics with the entire class.
    - Teams will be prepared to do Q&A with students and instructor.
    - All Teams will take a picture (smartphone) of their graphics and electronically submit to instructor/TA.
    - Each Team will turn in one Team Worksheet to instructor/TA.

6. Instructor will complete "Major Takeaways" with the class.

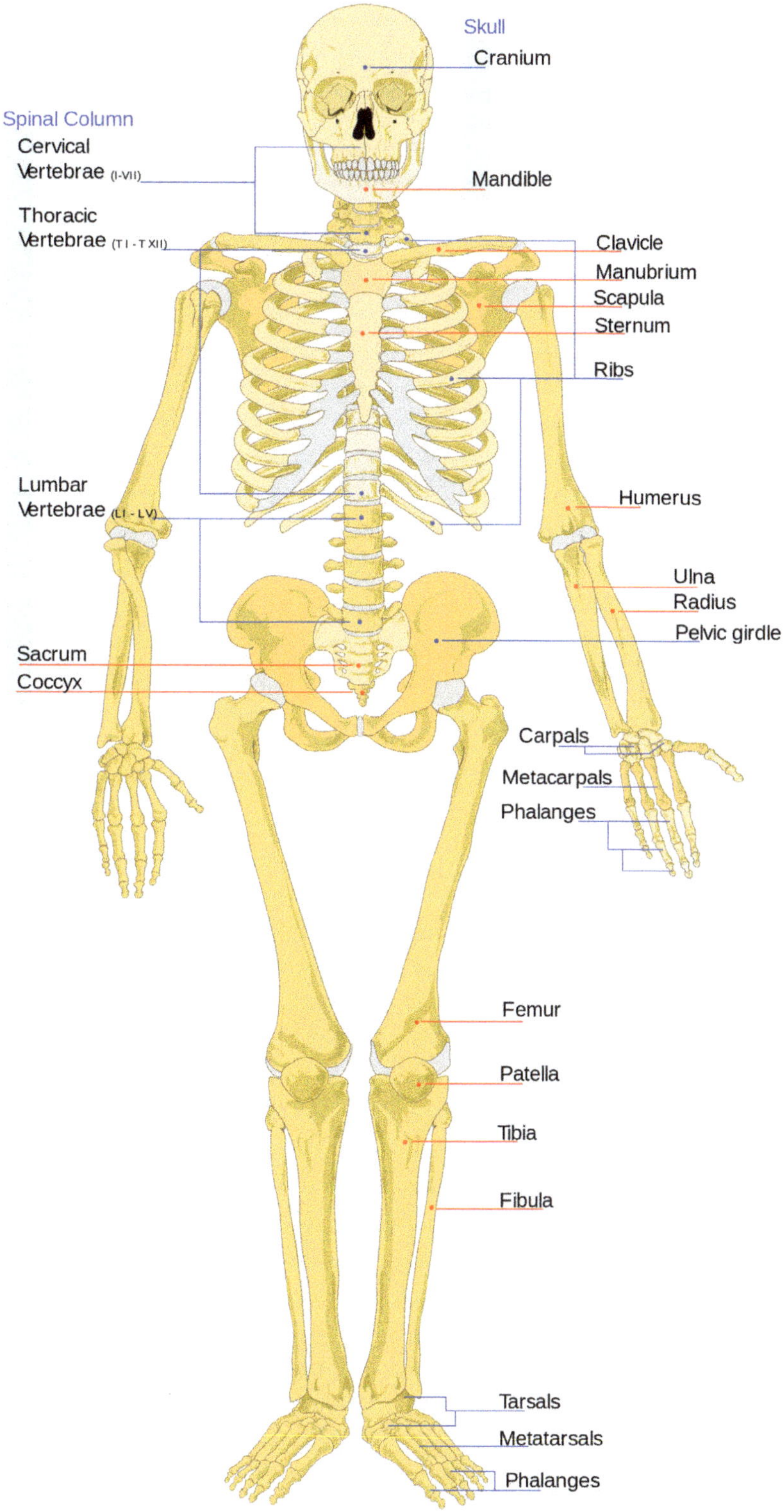

FIGURE 10.1 Skeleton front.

Novice students need to at least know all these major bones.

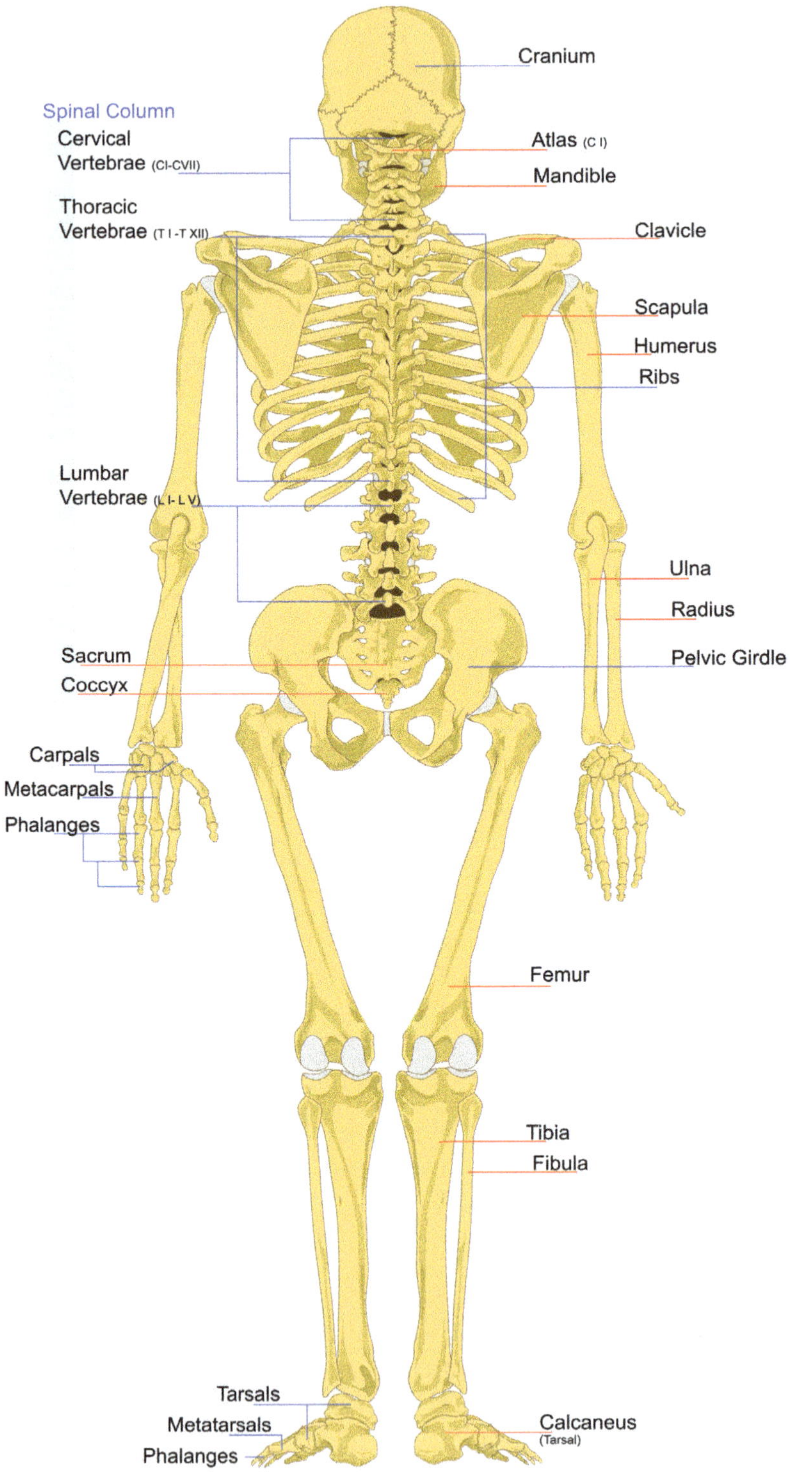

FIGURE 10.2 Skeleton back.

Introductory students need to at least know all these major bones.

Lab Team Worksheet

LAB 10—SKELETAL SYSTEM

Team Name: **Date:**

Team Members present for Lab:

1.

2.

3.

4.

Collaborating as a Team, answer the following questions. Each Team will turn in *one* Lab Team Worksheet at the completion of Lab.

1. What are the two conceptual functions of the skeleton? (See H_2O Sheet, chapter 2, *SS A&P*, 2nd Edition.)

____

____

2. The structural and functional unit of compact bone is the ______________.

3. List the four structures that make up the axial skeleton.

____

____

____

____

4. Bones are ______________ the way they are because of what they ______________.

5. The only bone in the body without any bone-to-bone articulation is the ______________.

Figure Credits

Fig. 10.1: Source: https://commons.wikimedia.org/wiki/File:Human_skeleton_front_en.svg.

Fig. 10.2: Source: https://commons.wikimedia.org/wiki/File:Human_skeleton_back_en.svg.

LAB 11

Homeostasis of Blood Calcium

Purpose of Lab and Desired Outcomes

Participate in Individual and Lab Team Activities to gain insight and understanding into the following topics:

1. Four areas where calcium balance is essential
2. Endocrine control of blood calcium levels
3. Calcium homeostasis—PTH and calcitonin
4. Three target organs of PTH and calcitonin

Pre-Lab Worksheet

LAB 11—CALCIUM HOMEOSTASIS AND BONE PHYSIOLOGY

Name: **Date:**

Each student will answer the following questions *before* coming to Lab.
Read chapter 10 (pages 126–129) in *SS A&P*, 2nd Edition or another reference regarding calcium homeostasis. Then, answer the following questions:

1. ______________________________ ***build*** bone by taking calcium from the blood and depositing it into the bone matrix.

2. ______________________________ ***chew*** bone by resorbing calcium from the bone matrix and transferring it into the blood.

3. Calcium homeostasis is essential for the normal function of what four areas?

   ____

   ____

   ____

   ____

4. PTH (parathyroid hormone) targets the following structures/organs:

   ____

   ____

   ____

   The endocrine hormone ______________________________ helps to lower blood calcium levels.

In-Lab Activities

1. Collection of student Pre-Lab Worksheets.
2. Instructor calls for QCs (Student Questions, Concerns, Confusions, and need for Clarification).
3. Instructor explanation of In-Lab Activities and desired outcomes from Lab time.
4. Follow the bullet points below to gain insight into calcium homeostasis.
    - Utilizing a blank sheet of standard notebook paper, each individual Lab Team member will draw, to the best of their ability, a conceptual diagram of calcium homeostasis.
    - Collaborate with each other while doing your individual drawings. Look stuff up online. *Help* each other. *Ask* each other questions. *Teach* each other.
    - Student drawings will be turned in to the instructor/TA for evaluation.
    - Each Team will then utilize a large sheet of paper or produce a graphic presentation (PPTs, Prezi, or Google Slides) of a conceptual diagram demonstrating calcium homeostasis.
5. Randomly selected (roll of the dice) Lab Teams will discuss graphics with the entire class.
    - Teams will be prepared to do Q&A with students and instructor.
    - All Teams will take a picture of their graphics (smartphone) and electronically submit it to instructor/TA.
    - Each Team will turn in one Team Worksheet to instructor/TA.
6. Instructor will complete "Major Takeaways" with the class.

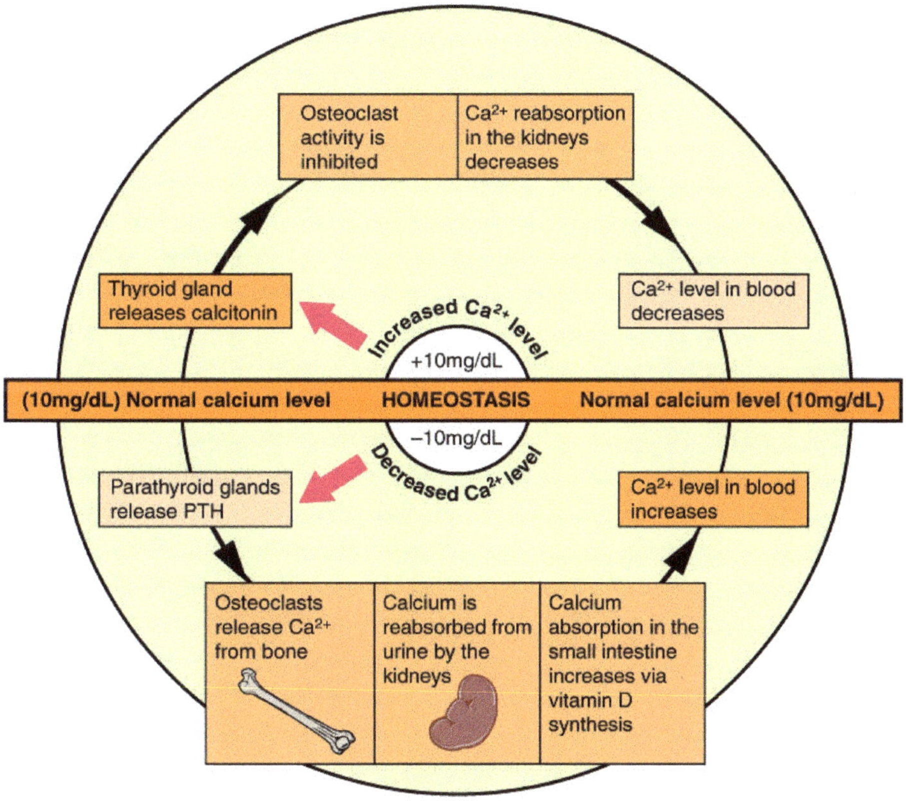

FIGURE 11.1 Simplistic flow chart of calcium homeostasis.

Graphic summarizing the processes maintaining the homeostatic balance of blood calcium.

Lab Team Worksheet

LAB 11—CALCIUM HOMEOSTASIS AND BONE PHYSIOLOGY

Team Name: **Date:**

Team Members present for Lab:

1.

2.

3.

4.

Collaborating as a Team, answer the following questions. Each Team will turn in *one* Lab Team Worksheet at the completion of Lab.

1. Negative feedback loops always ______________________ the original stimulus.

2. Positive feedback loops always ______________________ the original stimulus.

3. An ______________________ is the structural and functional unit of compact bone.

4. The neurotransmitter found at the NMJ of skeletal muscle is ________________ (abbreviated).

5. The neurotransmitter found at the NMJ of skeletal muscle is what primary type of biochemical?

   ____

6. The antagonistic endocrine hormone pair that maintains the homeostatic balance of blood calcium is

   ____

   ____

7. ______________________ is the "raw material" necessary for the body to manufacture vitamin D in the skin.

8. ______________________ is the ONLY vitamin that the human body can manufacture.

9. The ______________________ is the site of calcium storage inside muscle cells.

Figure Credit

Fig. 11.1: Copyright © by OpenStax College (CC by 3.0) at https://commons.wikimedia.org/wiki/File:625_Calcium_Homeostasis.jpg.

LAB 12

Skeletal Muscle System

Purpose of Lab and Desired Outcomes

Participate in Individual and Lab Team Activities to gain insight and understanding into the following topics:

1. Organizational patterns of skeletal muscle
2. Naming of skeletal muscles
3. Actions of muscles
4. Muscle pairs or groups—antagonistic or synergistic

Pre-Lab Worksheet

LAB 12—SKELETAL MUSCLE SYSTEM

Name: **Date:**

Complete the reading assignments for this Lab Activity. Then, answer the following questions:

1. The only *active* thing muscle can do is ______________________.

2. List the seven ways skeletal muscles are named.

____

____

____

____

____

____

____

3. The serratus anterior is also called the ______________________ muscle.

4. The sartorius is also called the ______________________ muscle.

In-Lab Activities

1. Collection of student Pre-Lab Worksheets.
2. Instructor calls for QCs (Student Questions, Concerns, Confusions, and need for Clarification).
3. Instructor explanation of In-Lab Activities and desired outcomes from Lab time.
4. Utilizing anatomical models, online resources, and pictures, student Teams will work collaboratively to identify the following skeletal muscles (listed superior to inferior):
   - Temporalis
   - Orbicularis oculi
   - Orbicularis oris
   - Platysma
   - Trapezius
   - Latissimus dorsi
   - Deltoid
   - Biceps brachii
   - Brachialis
   - Brachioradialis
   - Forearm flexors
   - Forearm extensors
   - Pectoralis major
   - Rhomboid major
   - Rhomboid minor
   - Supraspinatus
   - Infraspinatus
   - Teres minor
   - External oblique
   - Rectus abdominus
   - Internal oblique
   - Transversus abdominus
   - Quadriceps femoris
   - Biceps femoris
   - Semitendinosus
   - Semimembranosus
   - Sartorius
   - Tensor fascia lata
   - Gastrocnemius
   - Soleus
   - Tibialis anterior
5. While working to identify the above muscles, Teams will concurrently do the following:
   - On a large sheet of paper, draw a cross dividing the page into four equal squares, like windowpanes.
   - Draw an example of four of the major synergistic muscle groups from the list below in each of the four "panes." Or produce a graphic presentation (PPTs, Prezi, or Google Slides).

- Teams may choose any four from the list below:
    - Rotator cuff
    - Abdominal muscles
    - Flexors of the forearm at the elbow
    - Hamstrings
    - Calf muscles
- On a second large sheet of paper, Teams will draw out one of the antagonistic muscle pairs listed below. Or Teams will produce a graphic presentation (PPTs, Prezi, or Google Slides).
- Teams may choose any one pair from the list below:
    - Biceps and triceps brachii
    - Pectoralis major and minor
    - Quadriceps and hamstrings
- Teams will prepare to explain their graphics during class discussion time in #6.

6. Randomly selected (roll of the dice) Lab Teams will discuss graphics with the entire class.
    - Teams will be prepared to do Q&A with students and instructor.
    - All Teams will take a picture of their graphics (with a smartphone) and electronically submit it to instructor/TA.
    - Each Team will turn in one Team Worksheet to instructor/TA.
7. Instructor will complete "Major Takeaways" the class.

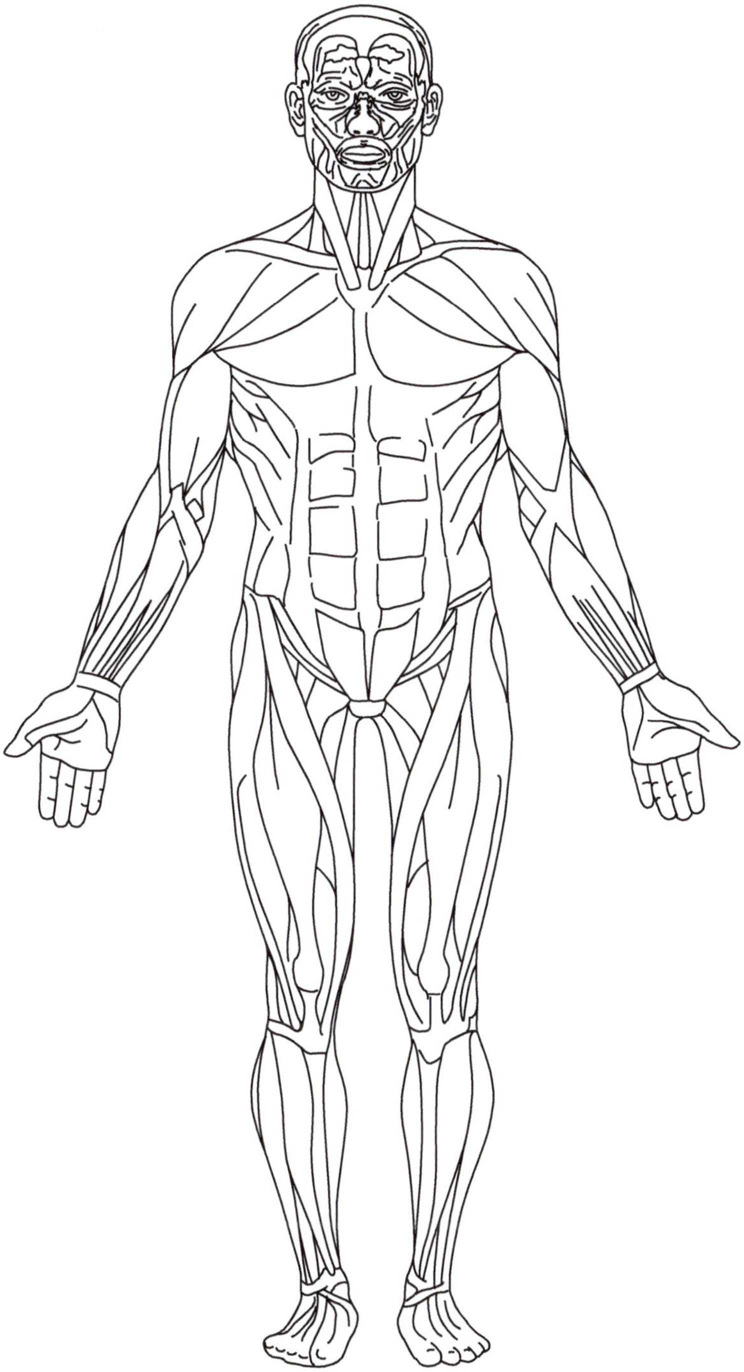

FIGURE 12.1 Coloring and labeling activity (anterior view).

Color and label the major muscles of importance for introductory-level learning.

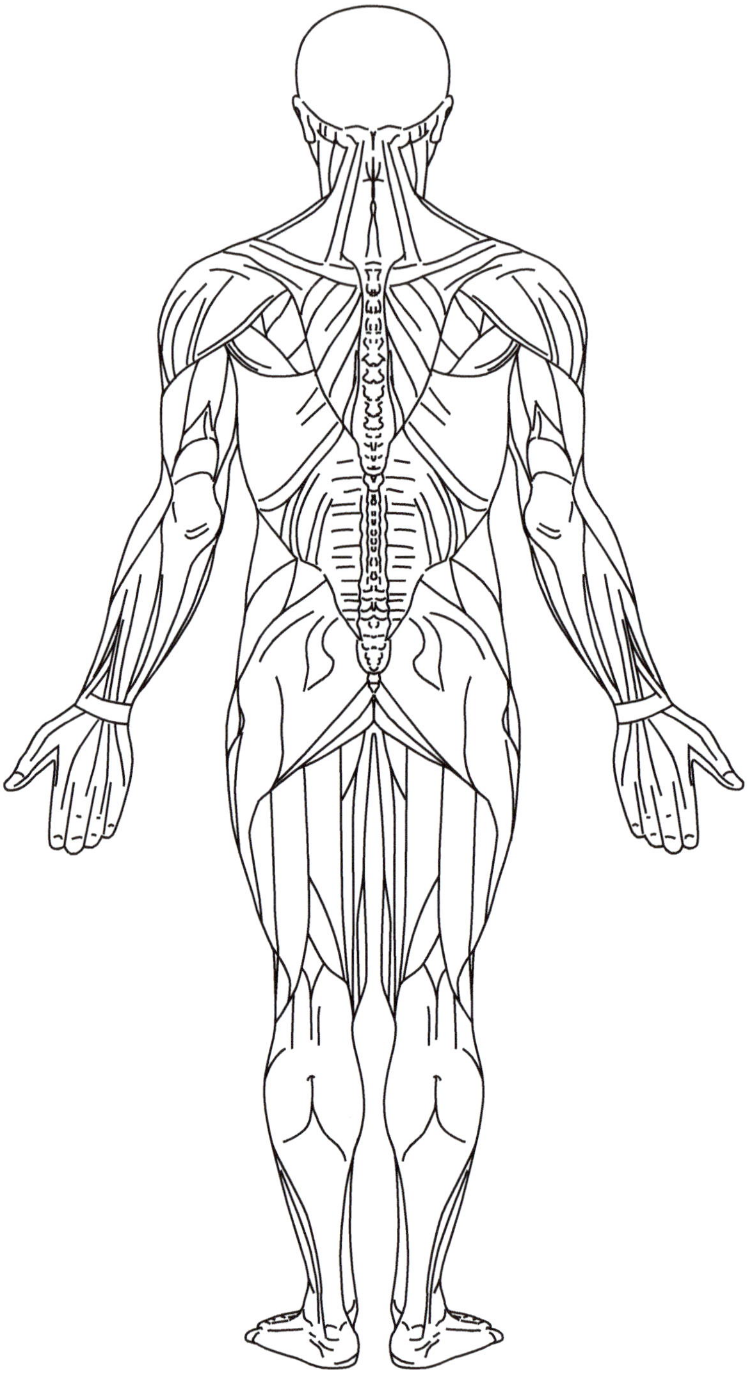

FIGURE 12.2 Coloring and labeling activity (posterior view).

Color and label the major muscles of importance for introductory-level learning.

Lab Team Worksheet

LAB 12—SKELETAL MUSCLE SYSTEM

Team Name: **Date:**

Team Members present for Lab:

1.

2.

3.

4.

Collaborating as a Team, answer the following questions. Each Team will turn in *one* Team Lab Worksheet at the completion of Lab.

1. Skeletal muscles are wrapped into groupings of three bundles, each surrounded by a connective tissue sheet. Name those sheets, starting with the most internal covering.

   ____

   ____

   ____

2. In the abdominal rectus muscle, the term *rectus* means ______________________________.

3. The ______________________________ of a muscle is the more stable or least movable part of the muscle.

4. List three muscles named based on the number of heads at their origin.

   ____

   ____

   ____

5. Muscles are ______________________ the way they are because of what they______________________.

Figure Credits

LAB 13

Skeletal Muscle Contraction

Purpose of Lab and Desired Outcomes

Participate in Individual and Lab Team Activities to gain insight and understanding into the following topics:

1. Structure of skeletal muscle
2. Neuromuscular junction
3. Importance of calcium and calcium homeostasis in muscle contraction
4. Sliding filament *theory* of contraction

Pre-Lab Worksheet

LAB 13—SKELETAL MUSCLE CONTRACTION

Name: **Date:**

Each student will answer the following questions *before* coming to Lab.

Part I. Go online and find the *Crash Course* (CC #21) YouTube video on muscle contraction. Listen, learn, and keep the CC website available in your browser to help you answer the following questions:

1. Muscle cells turn ______________________ potential energy into ______________________ energy

   and produce ______________________.

2. Muscle cells do two things. What are they?

   ______________________ (the only ACTIVE thing muscle can do)

   ______________________ (passive process)

3. Skeletal muscle is called "skeletal" because it attaches to ______________________. ("B" word maybe?)

4. Skeletal muscle has two other names. What are they?

   ____

   ____

5. A skeletal muscle is constructed like a "really sturdy" piece of ______________________. ("R" word)

6. The contractual units (protein molecules) of skeletal muscle, actin, and myosin are called

   ______________________.

Part II. Find an online animation of muscle contraction. This will help you understand muscle physiology as well as assist you when filling out the Lab Team Worksheet due at the end of Lab.

In-Lab Activities

1. Collection of student Pre-Lab Worksheets.
2. Instructor calls for QCs (Student Questions, Concerns, Confusions, and need for Clarification).
3. Instructor explanation of In-Lab Activities and desired outcomes from Lab time.
4. Follow the bullet points below to gain insight into muscle contraction.
   - Utilizing a blank sheet of standard notebook paper, each Lab Team member will draw, to the best of their ability, a conceptual diagram of skeletal muscle contraction. Or produce a graphic presentation (PPTs, Prezi, or Google Slides) of muscle contraction when in a virtual classroom environment.
   - Collaborate with each other while doing your drawings. Look stuff up online. *Help* each other. *Ask* each other questions. *Teach* each other.
   - Individual student drawings will be turned in to the instructor/TA for grading.
   - Each Team will then utilize a large sheet of paper and collaborate to draw a conceptual diagram of skeletal muscle contraction, including the NMJ and the sliding filament theory of contraction. Or produce a team graphic presentation (PPTs, Prezi, or Google Slides) of muscle contraction when in a virtual classroom environment.
5. Randomly selected (roll of the dice) Lab Teams will discuss graphics with the entire class.
   - Teams will be prepared to do Q&A with students and instructor.
   - All Teams will take a picture of their graphics and electronically submit it to instructor/TA.
   - Each Team will turn in one Team Worksheet to instructor/TA.
6. Instructor will complete "Major Takeaways" with the class.

Lab Team Worksheet

LAB 13—SKELETAL MUSCLE CONTRACTION

Team Name: **Date:**

Team Members present for Lab:

1.

2.

3.

4.

Collaborating as a Team, answer the following questions. Each Team will turn in *one* Lab Team Worksheet at the completion of Lab.

1. The only *active* thing a muscle can do is ______________________________.
2. ______________________________ is a cation essential for muscle contraction.
3. A single somatic motor neuron and all the muscle fibers (cells) it innervates is called a ______________________________.
4. A ______________________________ is the contractile unit of a muscle.
5. The neurotransmitter found at the NMJ of skeletal muscle is ______________________ (abbreviated).
6. Energy for muscle contraction is supplied by ______________________________.
7. The specialized region of the sarcolemma, which has folds and is covered by the synaptic knob of the motor neuron, is called the ______________________________.
8. ______________________________ is the current theory explaining the contraction of skeletal muscle.
9. The ______________________________ is the site of calcium storage inside muscle cells.
10. The amount of additional oxygen that must be inhaled following exercise to restore pre-exercise conditions is called ______________________________.

LAB 14

Nervous System Anatomy

Purpose of Lab and Desired Outcomes

Participate in Individual and Lab Team Activities to gain insight and understanding into the following topics:

1. Organizational structure of the nervous system (NS)
2. Structure of a neuron
3. Structural and functional classification of neurons
4. Major structures of the CNS—brain and spinal cord
5. Cranial nerves
6. Spinal nerves
7. Major peripheral nerves
8. Major structures of the eye and ear

Pre-Lab Worksheet

LAB 14—NERVOUS SYSTEM

Name: **Date:**

Each student will answer the following questions *before* coming to Lab:

1. The structural and functional unit of the nervous system (NS) is the ______________________.

2. List the three parts of a neuron.

   ____

   ____

   ____

3. The most common neuroglial cell is the ______________________.

4. List the three structural types of neurons.

   ____

   ____

   ____

5. The most common functional type of neuron is the ______________________ neuron.

6. Sensory neurons are also known as ______________________ neurons.

In-Lab Activities

1. Collection of student Pre-Lab Worksheets.
2. Instructor calls for QCs (Student Questions, Concerns, Confusions, and need for Clarification).
3. Instructor explanation of In-Lab Activities and desired outcomes from Lab time.
4. Utilizing anatomical models, online resources, and pictures, student Teams will work collaboratively to identify the following structures of the nervous system (NS).
    - Cranium and brain
        - Meninges—pia mater, arachnoid mater, dura mater
        - Ventricles of the brain—1—4
            - Choroid plexus
            - Cerebral aqueduct
        - Lobes of the brain
            - Frontal
            - Parietal
            - Temporal
            - Occipital
            - Insula
    - Midsagittal section of the brain
        - Cerebral lobes
            - Frontal
            - Parietal
            - Occipital
        - Central sulcus
        - Corpus callosum
        - Thalamus
        - Hypothalamus
        - Cerebrum
        - Midbrain
        - Pons
        - Medulla oblongata
        - Cerebellum
    - Cranial nerve origins
        - Inferior view of the brain
        - CN I–XII
    - Spinal cord (SC)
        - X-section of SC
        - White matter
            - Dorsal columns
            - Lateral columns
            - Ventral columns

    - Gray matter
        - Dorsal horn
        - Lateral horn
        - Ventral horn
    - Central canal
    - Dorsal root
    - Dorsal root ganglion
    - Ventral root
- Eye
    - Extraocular muscles (skeletal)
        - Rectus—four muscles
        - Obliques—two muscles
    - Cornea
    - Iris
    - Pupil
    - Sclera
    - Choroid
    - Retina
    - Optic disc
- Ear
    - Outer ear
        - Pinna—auricle
        - External auditory canal
    - Tympanic membrane
    - Middle ear or tympanic cavity
        - Malleus
        - Incus
        - Stapes
    - Inner ear
        - Cochlea—organ of hearing
        - Vestibule
        - Semicircular canals
        - CN VIII—vestibulocochlear
          Vestibular nerve
          Cochlear nerve

While working to identify the above structures, Teams will concurrently do the following:

- On a large sheet of paper, draw a horizontal line across the sheet dividing it into equal top and bottom halves.
- Draw a graphic of the eye in the top half of the page and a graphic of the ear in the bottom half of the sheet. Or produce a graphic presentation (PPTs, Prezi, or Google Slides) of the eye and the ear when in a virtual classroom environment. On another large sheet of paper, Teams will draw

out a flow chart showing the organization of the NS as demonstrated in Figure 12.1 in *SS A&P*, 2nd Edition. Or produce a graphic presentation (PPTs, Prezi, or Google Slides) of the flow chart when in a virtual classroom environment.

- Teams will prepare to explain their graphics during class discussion time in #5.

5. Randomly selected (roll of the dice) Lab Teams will discuss their graphics with the entire class by leading a class discussion.
   - Teams will be prepared to do Q&A with students and instructor.
   - All Teams will take a picture (with a smartphone) of their flip chart graphics and electronically submit it to instructor/TA.
   - Each Team will turn in one Team Worksheet to instructor/TA.
6. Instructor will complete "Major Takeaways" with the class.

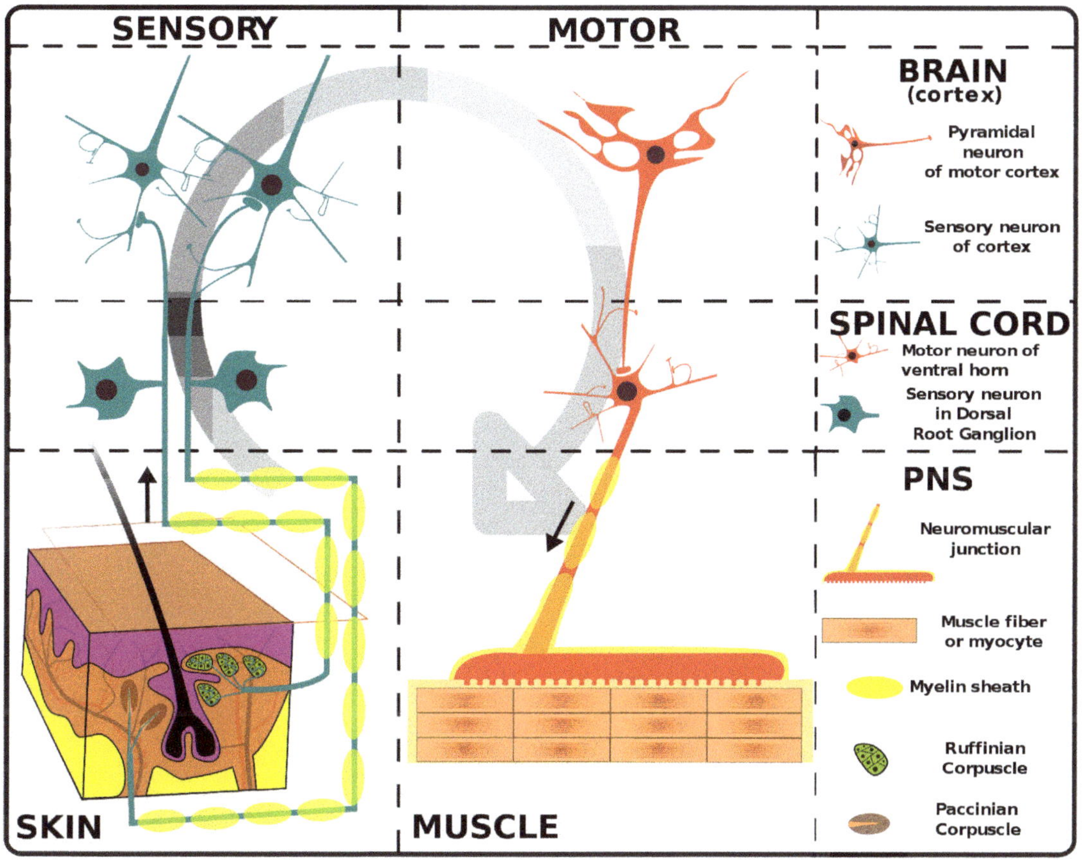

FIGURE 14.1 Simplistic, conceptual overview of nervous system structure/function.

Compare the functional and structural types of neurons (Figure 12.4 in *SS A&P* text, 2nd Edition).

Lab Team Worksheet

LAB 14—NERVOUS SYSTEM

Team Name: **Date:**

Team Members present for Lab:

1.

2.

3.

4.

Collaborating as a Team, answer the following questions. Each Team will turn in *one* Lab Team Worksheet at the completion of Lab.

1. Peripheral nerves are wrapped into groupings of three bundles each surrounded by a connective tissue sheet. Name those sheets, starting with the most internal covering.

____

____

____

2. List the four neuroglial cells located in the CNS.

____

____

____

____

3. List the two neuroglial cells located in the PNS.

____

____

4. ____________________ are accumulations of ependymal cells in the ventricles of the brain that produce cerebral spinal fluid (CSF).

Figure Credit

Fig. 14.1: Copyright © by Looie496 (CC BY-SA 3.0) at https://commons.wikimedia.org/wiki/File:Nervous_system_organization_en.svg.

LAB 15

Nervous System—Action Potential

Purpose of Lab and Desired Outcomes

Participate in Individual and Lab Team Activities to gain insight and understanding into the following topics:

1. Organization of the nervous system (NS)
2. Resting membrane potential
3. Sodium potassium pump theory
4. Action potential—depolarization and repolarization
5. Myelin sheaths and saltatory conduction

Pre-Lab Worksheet

LAB 15—NERVOUS SYSTEM—ACTION POTENTIAL

Name: **Date:**

Each student will answer the following questions *before* coming to Lab:

1. The NS (nervous system) is the body's ____________________ system.

2. The NS functions ____________________. (How?)

3. The ES (endocrine system) functions ____________________. (How?)

4. The ____________________ is the structural and functional unit of the NS.

5. List the three major parts (components) of a neuron.

____

____

____

6. In theory, the resting membrane potential (RMP) is maintained by what pump?

____

7. An action potential (AP) sending an electrical impulse down an axon is caused by what two events?

____

____

In-Lab Activities

1. Collection of student Pre-Lab Worksheets.
2. Instructor calls for QCs (Student Questions, Concerns, Confusions, and need for Clarification).
3. Instructor explanation of In-Lab Activities and desired outcomes from Lab time.
4. Follow the bullet points below to gain insight into an action potential.
   - Utilizing a blank sheet of standard notebook paper, each Lab Team member will draw the organization flow chart of the NS found in Figure 12.1 in *SS A&P*, 2nd Edition. Or produce a graphic presentation (PPTs, Prezi, or Google Slides) of an action potential when in a virtual classroom environment.
   - On the back of the same sheet, or a second large sheet of paper, Team members will draw a graphic representation of an action potential (AP). Or produce a graphic presentation (PPTs, Prezi, or Google Slides) of an action potential when in a virtual classroom environment.
   - Collaborate with each other while doing your individual drawings. Look stuff up online. *Help* each other. *Ask* each other questions. *Teach* each other.
   - Individual student drawings will be turned in to the instructor/TA for grading.
   - Each Team will then utilize a full sheet collaborating to draw a conceptual diagram of an action potential (AP), including RMP, depolarization, repolarization, and return to RMP. Or produce a graphic presentation (PPTs, Prezi, or Google Slides) of an action potential when in a virtual classroom environment.
5. Randomly selected (roll of the dice) Lab Teams will discuss their graphics with the entire class.
   - Teams will be prepared to do Q&A with students and instructor.
   - All Teams will take a picture of their graphics and electronically submit it to instructor/TA.
   - Each Team will turn in one Team Worksheet to instructor/TA.
6. Instructor will complete "Major Takeaways" with the class.

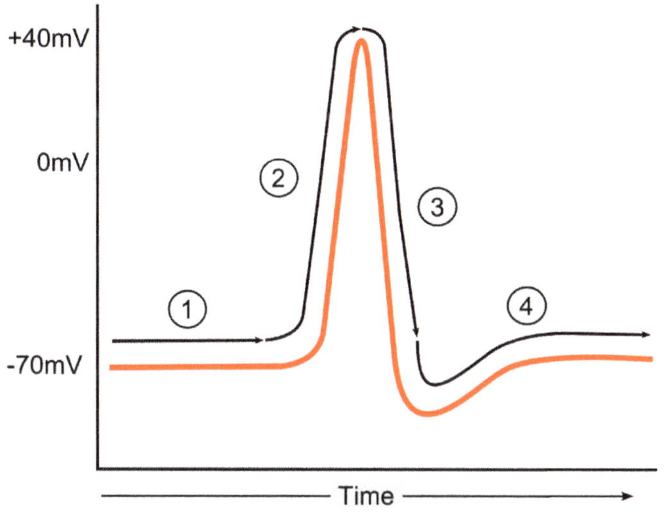

FIGURE 15.1 What do the numbers on this AP represent?

Label the four phases of an action potential.

Lab Team Worksheet

LAB 15—NERVOUS SYSTEM—ACTION POTENTIAL

Team Name: **Date:**

Team members present for Lab:

1.

2.

3.

4.

Collaborating as a Team, answer the following questions. Each Team will turn in *one* Lab Team Worksheet at the completion of Lab.

1. In the sodium-potassium pump theory, ______________ sodium ions are pumped out of the neuron for every ______________ potassium ions pumped into the neuron.

2. Large ______________ anions that are trapped inside the neuron also contribute to the RMP.

3. In an action potential (AP), depolarization is caused by sodium ions moving from ______________ space to ______________ space by the process of ______________.

4. In an action potential (AP), repolarization is caused by ______________ ions moving from ______________ space to ______________ space by the process of ______________.

Figure Credit

LAB 16

Nervous System—Synapse

Purpose of Lab and Desired Outcomes

Participate in Individual and Lab Team activities to gain insight and understanding into the following topics:

1. Organization of the nervous system (NS)
2. Synapses—electrical and chemical
3. Chemical synapse structure
4. Chemical synapse function

Pre-Lab Worksheet

LAB 16—NERVOUS SYSTEM—SYNAPSE

Name: **Date:**

Each student will answer the following questions *before* coming to Lab:

1. The NS structure that allows an impulse to pass from one neuron to another neuron is called a

   ______________________________.

2. List the two types of synapses.

   ____

   ____

3. The neuron that is located prior to a synapse is the ______________________________ neuron.

4. The neuron that is located after a synapse is ______________________________ neuron.

5. The ______________________________ is the space between the two neurons comprising a synapse.

6. ______________________________ is the cation essential for the release of a neurotransmitter (NT) from the presynaptic neuron.

7. Neurotransmitters are produced by ____.

8. List two common neurotransmitters; you can include the NT found at the NMJ of skeletal muscle.

   ____

   ____

In-Lab Activities

1. Collection of student Pre-Lab Worksheets.
2. Instructor calls for QCs (Student Questions, Concerns, Confusions, and need for Clarification).
3. Instructor explanation of In-Lab Activities and desired outcomes from Lab time.
4. Follow the bullet points below to gain insight into a chemical synapse.
   - Utilizing a blank sheet of standard notebook paper, each Lab Team member will draw a graphic of a chemical synapse. Or produce a graphic presentation (PPTs, Prezi, or Google Slides) of a chemical synapse when in a virtual classroom environment.
   - On the back of the same sheet, or on a separate sheet, Team members will draw a graphic representation of an electrical synapse. Or produce a graphic presentation (PPTs, Prezi, or Google Slides) of an electrical synapse when in a virtual classroom environment.
   - Collaborate with each other while doing your drawings. Look stuff up online. *Help* each other. *Ask* each other questions. *Teach* each other.
   - Student drawings will be turned in to the instructor/TA for grading.
   - Each Team will then utilize a full sheet of paper collaborating to draw a conceptual diagram of a chemical synapse. Or produce a graphic presentation (PPTs, Prezi, or Google Slides) of a chemical synapse when in a virtual classroom environment.
5. Randomly selected (roll of the dice) Lab Teams will discuss graphics with the entire class.
   - Teams will be prepared to do Q&A with students and instructor.
   - All Teams will take a picture of their graphics and electronically submit it to instructor/TA.
   - Each Team will turn in one Team Worksheet to instructor/TA.
6. Instructor will complete "Major Takeaways" with the class.

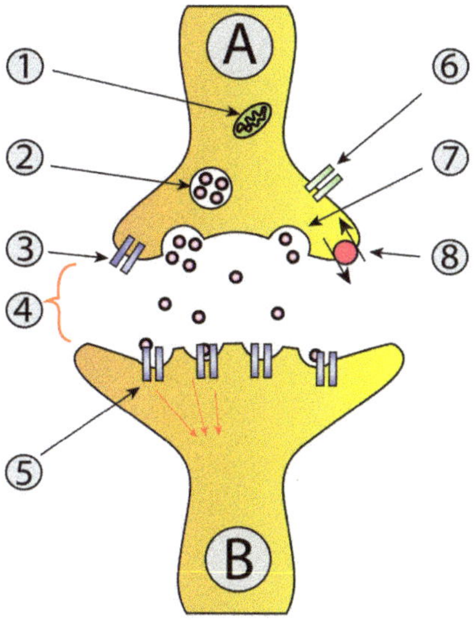

FIGURE 16.1 Chemical synapse identification opportunity (#3 is an autoreceptor and #8 is a reuptake pump).

Label the eight structures of a chemical synapse.

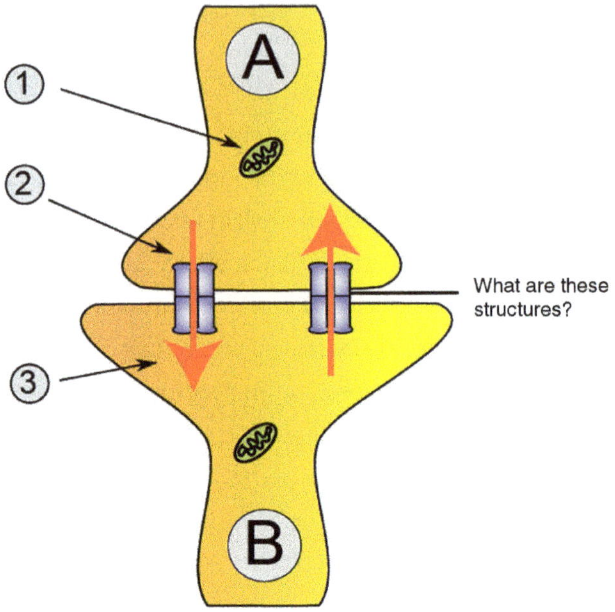

FIGURE 16.2 Electrical synapse identification opportunity.

What is the difference between an electrical synapse and a chemical synapse?

Lab Team Worksheet

LAB 16—NERVOUS SYSTEM—SYNAPSE

Team Name: **Date:**

Team members present for Lab:

1.

2.

3.

4.

Collaborating as a Team, answer the following questions. Each Team will turn in *one* Lab Team Worksheet at the completion of Lab.

1. The most common synapse in the NS is the ______________________ synapse.

2. List the three main components of a chemical synapse.

   ____

   ____

   ____

3. Neurotransmitters (NTs), like ACh and serotonin, are produced by the presynaptic neuron through the process of ______________________ ______________________.

4. An ________________ traveling down the presynaptic neuron causes ________________ protein channels to open, allowing ________________ ions to rush down their concentration gradient into the cell.

5. The influx of calcium ions into the presynaptic neuron causes the release of the NT through the process of ______________________.

6. The NT crosses the synaptic cleft and docks with ______________________ integral proteins, which open and allow sodium ions to rush into the postsynaptic neuron, causing depolarization creating an AP.

Figure Credits

LAB 17

Endocrine System

Purpose of Lab and Desired Outcomes

Participate in Individual and Lab Team Activities to gain insight and understanding into the following topics:

1. Homeostasis—conceptual function of the endocrine system
2. Concept of negative feedback loops
3. Thyroid hormone homeostasis
4. Glucose homeostasis
5. Calcium homeostasis

Pre-Lab Worksheet

LAB 17—ENDOCRINE SYSTEM

Name: **Date:**

Each student will answer the following questions *before* coming to Lab.

Go online and find the *Crash Course* YouTube video on endocrine function. Listen, learn, and keep the CC website available in your browser to help you answer the following questions:

1. The body's chemical "communication" system is the ______________________ system.

2. List three steroid-based hormones.

 ____

 ____

 ____

3. List four nonsteroidal endocrine hormones.

 ____

 ____

 ____

 ____

4. A negative feedback loop always ______________________ the original stimulus.

5. A positive feedback loop always ______________________ the original stimulus.

In-Lab Activities

1. Collection of student Pre-Lab Worksheets.
2. Instructor calls for QCs (Student Questions, Concerns, Confusions, and need for Clarification).
3. Instructor explanation of In-Lab Activities and desired outcomes from Lab time.
4. Follow the bullet points below to gain insight into endocrine function.
   - Utilizing a blank sheet of standard notebook paper, each Lab Team member will draw, to the best of their ability, a conceptual diagram of a negative feedback loop. Or produce a digital presentation (Google Slides, PPTs, or Prezi) demonstrating negative feedback loops.
   - Collaborate with each other while doing your drawings. Look stuff up online. *Help* each other. *Ask* each other questions. *Teach* each other.
   - Student drawings will be turned in to the instructor/TA for grading.
   - Each Team will then utilize a full sheet of paper collaborating to draw a conceptual diagram of the negative feedback loops involved in the regulation of thyroid hormone. Or teams will produce a digital presentation (Google Slides, PPTs, or Prezi) demonstrating negative feedback loops for thyroid hormone.
5. Randomly selected (roll of the dice) Lab Teams will lead a discussion of their graphics with the entire class.
   - Teams will be prepared to do Q&A with students and instructor.
   - All Teams will take a picture of their graphics and electronically submit it to instructor/TA.
   - Each Team will turn in one Team Worksheet to instructor/TA.
6. Instructor will complete "Major Takeaways" with the class.

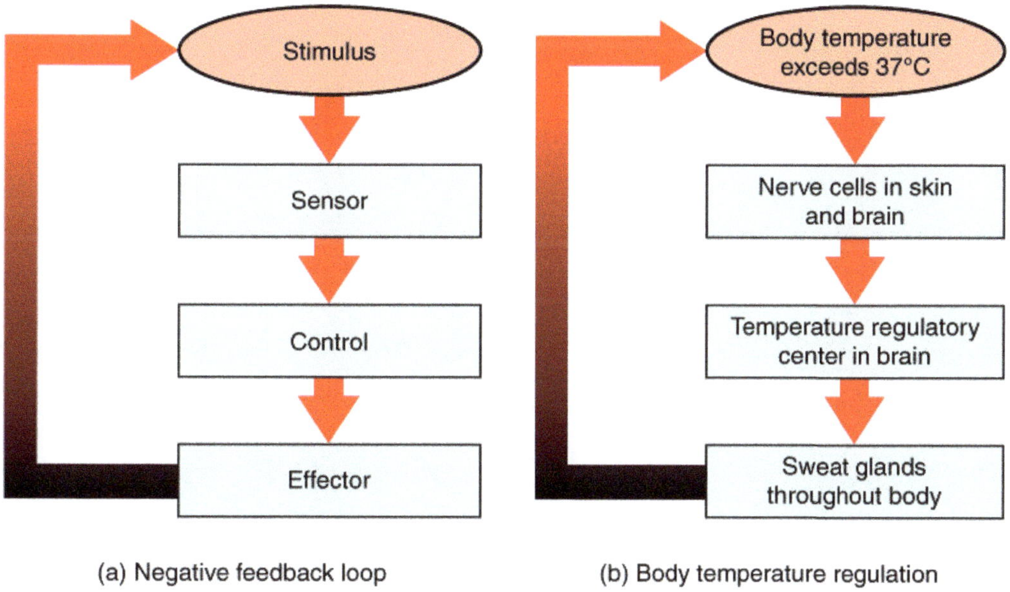

FIGURE 17.1 Remember, a negative feedback loop always reverses the original stimulus.

Conceptual diagram of a negative feedback loop.

Lab Team Worksheet

LAB 17—ENDOCRINE SYSTEM

Team Name: **Date:**

Team Members present for Lab:

1.

2.

3.

4.

Collaborating as a Team, answer the following questions. Each Team will turn in *one* Lab Team Worksheet at the completion of Lab.

1. The endocrine system communicates ______________________.

2. A negative feedback loop always ______________________ the original stimulus.

3. A positive feedback loops always ______________________ the original stimulus.

4. The ______________________ gland is the master endocrine gland.

5. List four endocrine hormones that are proteins.

____

____

____

____

6. List two steroid-based endocrine hormones.

____

____

Figure Credit

LAB 18

CVS—Cardiovascular System—Anatomy

Purpose of Lab and Desired Outcomes

Participate in Individual and Lab Team Activities to gain insight and understanding into the following topics:

1. Organization of the human CVS
2. CVS Flow Chart (Figure 14.1—*SS A&P* text, 2nd Edition)
3. Gross anatomy of the heart
    - Anterior view
    - Posterior view
    - Internal view

Pre-Lab Worksheet

LAB 18—CVS—CARDIOVASCULAR SYSTEM—HEART

Name: **Date:**

Complete the reading assignments for this Lab Activity. Then, answer the following questions. Refer to the CVS Flow Chart (Figure 14.1 in *SS A&P* text, 2nd Edition).

1. The CVS (cardiovascular system) is the body's ____________________ system.

2. Conceptually, what are the three divisions of a "typical" transportation system?

   ____

   ____

   ____

3. Conceptually, what are the three divisions of the CVS?

   ____

   ____

   ____

4. The heart is ____________________ the way it is because of what it ____________________.

5. Heart chambers that receive blood are called ____________________.

In-Lab Activities

1. Collection of student Pre-Lab Worksheets.
2. Instructor calls for QCs (Student Questions, Concerns, Confusions, and need for Clarification).
3. Instructor explanation of In-Lab Activities and desired outcomes from Lab time.
4. Utilizing anatomical models, online resources, and pictures, student Teams will work collaboratively to identify the following structures of the CVS:
   - **Anterior heart**
     - Superior vena cava
     - Inferior vena cava
     - Pulmonary trunk
     - Left and right pulmonary artery
     - Right auricle
     - Right atrium
     - Aorta
       1. Ascending
       2. Arch
       3. Descending
     - Branches of the ascending aorta
       1. Left coronary artery
          Circumflex artery
          Anterior interventricular (left anterior descending) artery
       2. Right coronary artery
     - Branches of the arch of the aorta
       1. Brachiocephalic trunk
       2. Left common carotid artery
       3. Left subclavian artery
     - Ligamentum arteriosum
   - **Posterior heart**
     - Aorta
     - Left pulmonary artery
     - Auricle of left atrium
     - Left atrium
     - Left pulmonary veins
     - Coronary sinus
     - Apex of heart
     - Inferior vena cava
     - Right pulmonary veins
     - Right pulmonary artery
     - Superior vena cava

- **Internal heart**
    - Aorta
    - Superior vena cava
    - Pulmonary trunk
    - Right pulmonary veins
    - Right atrium
    - Fossa ovalis
    - Tricuspid valve
    - Right ventricle
    - Chordae tendineae
    - Inferior vena cava
    - Endocardium
    - Myocardium
    - Epicardium
    - Interventricular septum
    - Papillary muscle
    - Left ventricle
    - Pulmonary semilunar valve
    - Aortic semilunar valve
    - Bicuspid (mitral) valve
    - Left pulmonary veins
    - Left atrium
    - Left pulmonary artery

While working to identify the above structures, Teams will concurrently do the following:

- On a large sheet of paper, draw out a graphic picture of an internal view of the heart labeling the structures listed above. Or produce a digital presentation (Google Slides, PPTs, or Prezi) demonstrating the internal anatomy of the heart.
- On a second large sheet of paper, Teams will draw out a graphic flow chart showing the flow of blood through the heart, out to the lungs, back to the heart, out to the body, and then back to the right side of the heart. Or produce a digital presentation (Google Slides, PPTs, or Prezi) demonstrating blood flow through the heart.
- Teams will prepare to explain their graphics during class discussion time in #5 below.

5. Randomly selected (roll of the dice) Lab Teams will lead a class discussion of the graphics.
    - Teams will be prepared to do Q&A with students and instructor.
    - All Teams will take a picture of their graphics and electronically submit it to instructor/TA.
    - Each Team will turn in one Team Worksheet to instructor/TA.
6. Instructor will complete "Major Takeaways" with the class.

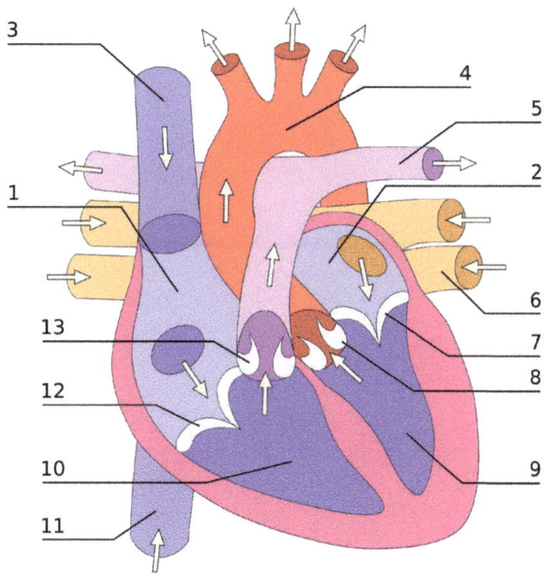

FIGURE 18.1 Labeling opportunity for the heart (internal view).

Label all thirteen structures and review blood flow through the heart.

Lab Team Worksheet

LAB 18—CVS—CARDIOVASCULAR SYSTEM—HEART

Team Name: **Date:**

Team Members present for Lab:

1.

2.

3.

4.

Collaborating as a Team, answer the following questions. Each Team will turn in *one* Lab Team Worksheet at the completion of Lab. Refer to the CVS Flow Chart, Figure 14.1 in *SS A&P*, 2nd Edition.

1. Vessels that always carry blood away from the heart are called ______________________.

2. Vessels that always carry blood toward the heart are called ______________________.

3. Veins have ______________________, which maintain a one-way flow of blood.

4. Arteries are ______________________-______________________; veins are not.

5. Arteries are ____________________ the way they are because of what they ________________.

6. The ______________________ is the largest artery in the body.

7. The vessel that drains venous blood from the myocardium into the right atrium is called the ______________________ ______________________.

8. ______________________ are where the "work" gets done in the CVS.

9. Gap junctions form the histologically identifying characteristic of cardiac muscle called ______________________ ______________________.

Figure Credit

LAB 19

CVS—Cardiovascular System—Vessels

Purpose of Lab and Desired Outcomes

Participate in Individual and Lab Team Activities to gain insight and understanding into the following topics:

1. Organization of the human cardiovascular system (CVS)
2. CVS Flow Chart (Figure 14.1 *SS A&P* text, 2nd Edition)
3. Gross anatomy of the major vessels
    - Arteries
    - Veins

Pre-Lab Worksheet

LAB 19—CVS—CARDIOVASCULAR SYSTEM—VESSELS

Name: **Date:**

Complete the reading assignments for this Lab Activity. Then answer the following questions. Refer to the CVS Flow Chart (Figure 14.1 in *SS A&P*).

1. The CVS (cardiovascular system) is the body's ____________________ system.

2. The ____________________ is the largest artery in the body.

3. What are the two branches of the *ascending* aorta?

____

____

4. The aorta is ____________________ the way it is because of what it ____________________.

5. List the three branches of the arch of the aorta, proximal to distal.

____

____

____

6. ____________________ are where the "work" gets done in the CVS.

In-Lab Activities

1. Collection of student Pre-Lab Worksheets.
2. Instructor calls for QCs (Student Questions, Concerns, Confusions, and need for Clarification).
3. Instructor explanation of In-Lab Activities and desired outcomes from Lab time.
4. Utilizing anatomical models, online resources, and pictures, student Teams will work collaboratively to identify the following vascular structures of the CVS.
    - With few exceptions, deep veins of the body parallel the deep arteries—so learn the arteries. Where there's a deep artery, there's usually a deep vein by the same name running parallel to the artery! **CONCEPTS simplify learning!**
    - Understand how arteries and veins are named.
        - Area of the body—axillary, femoral, etc.
        - Organ supplied or drained—gastric, digital, hepatic.
    - **MAJOR VESSELS of the heart**
        - Superior vena cava
        - Inferior vena cava
        - Pulmonary trunk
        - Pulmonary veins
        - Aorta
        - Left and right coronary arteries—plus anterior descending
        - Coronary sinus
    - **MAJOR ARTERIES of the body**
        - Brachiocephalic trunk
        - Left common carotid artery
        - Left subclavian artery
        - Internal carotid arteries (left and right)
        - External carotid arteries (left and right)
        - Axillary arteries (left and right)
        - Brachial arteries (left and right)
        - Ulnar arteries (left and right)
        - Radial arteries (left and right)
        - Palmar arch (left and right)
        - Digital arteries (left and right)
        - Descending aorta
        - Abdominal aorta
            - Celiac trunk
              Gastric artery
              Splenic artery
              Hepatic artery
            - Superior mesenteric artery
            - Renal arteries (left and right)
            - Gonadal arteries (ovarian and testicular)

        - Inferior mesenteric artery
        - Common iliac arteries (terminal branches of the abdominal aorta)
          Left
          Right
        - Internal iliac arteries (left and right)
        - External iliac arteries (left and right)
        - Femoral arteries (left and right)
        - Deep femoral arteries (left and right)
        - Popliteal arteries (left and right)
        - Tibial arteries (left and right)
          Anterior
          Posterior
        - Plantar arch (left and right)
        - Digital arteries (left and right)
- **DEEP VEINS of the body**
    - REMEMBER—deep veins usually parallel deep arteries
        - For example:
          Subclavian artery—subclavian vein
          Axillary artery—axillary vein
          Femoral artery—femoral vein
        - If you focus on learning the deep arteries, then you also know most of the deep veins
    - Exceptions of parallel artery/vein concept
        - Superior and inferior vena cava
        - Common carotid and internal jugular vein
        - Deep femoral—no parallel vein
        - Azygos and hemiazygos veins
- **HEPATIC PORTAL SYSTEM—essential to know**
    - Veins drain blood rich with nutrients from the GI tract.
        - Splenic vein
        - Superior mesenteric vein
        - Inferior mesenteric vein
    - The three veins above drain into the hepatic portal vein, which drains into the liver.

While working to identify the above structures, Teams will concurrently do the following:

- On a large sheet of paper, draw out a graphic of the hepatic portal system. Or produce a digital presentation (Google Slides, PPTs, or Prezi) demonstrating the hepatic portal system.
- Teams will prepare to explain their graphic during class discussion time in #5 below.

5. Randomly selected (roll of the dice) Lab Teams will lead a class discussion about their graphic.
    - Teams will be prepared to do Q&A with students and instructor.
    - All Teams will take a picture of their graphics and electronically submit it to instructor/TA.
    - Each Team will turn in one Team Worksheet to instructor/TA.
6. Instructor will complete "Major Takeaways" with the class.

Lab Team Worksheet

LAB 19—CVS—CARDIOVASCULAR SYSTEM—VESSELS

Team Name: **Date:**

Team Members present for Lab:

1.

2.

3.

4.

Collaborating as a Team, answer the following questions. Each Team will turn in *one* Lab Team Worksheet at the completion of Lab. Refer to the CVS Flow Chart (Figure 14.1 in *SS A&P*, 2nd Edition).

1. Vessels that always carry blood away from the heart are called ______________________.

2. Vessels that always carry blood toward the heart are called ______________________.

3. Veins have ______________________, which maintain a one-way flow of blood.

4. Arteries are ________________ the way they are because of what they ________________.

5. The ______________________ is the largest artery in the body.

6. The vessel that drains venous blood from the myocardium into the right atrium is called the

   ______________________ ______________________.

7. ______________________ are where the "work" gets done in the CVS.

8. The subclavian artery is located inferior to the ______________________.

LAB 20

CVS—Blood Flow through the Heart

Purpose of Lab and Desired Outcomes

Participate in Individual and Lab Team Activities to gain insight and understanding into the following topics:

1. Anatomical structure of the heart and great vessels
2. Electrical stimulation of the heart
3. Blood flow through the heart, to the lungs, back to the heart, out to the body, and back to the heart
4. Blood turbulence

Pre-Lab Worksheet

LAB 20—BLOOD FLOW THROUGH THE HEART/BLOOD TURBULENCE

Name: **Date:**

Complete reading assignments for this lab activity. Figure 14.1 in *SS A&P*, 2nd Edition will be helpful. Then, answer the following questions:

1. The CVS is the body's ______________________ system.

2. A transportation system has three main components. List them below.

 ____

 ____

 ____

3. The ______________________ is the CVS engine providing energy to move blood.

4. List the four chambers of the heart, receiving chambers first, then ejection chambers.

 ____

 ____

 ____

 ____

5. Conceptually, any sound, other than S1 and S2, is caused by ______________________.

In-Lab Activities

1. Collection of student Pre-Lab Worksheets.
2. Instructor calls for QCs (Student Questions, Concerns, Confusions, and need for Clarification).
3. Instructor explanation of In-Lab Activities and desired outcomes from Lab time.
4. Follow the bullet points below to gain insight into cardiac function.
   - Utilizing a blank sheet of standard notebook paper, each Lab Team member will draw a graphic of the internal heart structure and indicate the flow of blood through the heart. The diagram must indicate oxygenated (red) and deoxygenated (blue) blood. Or produce a digital presentation (Google Slides, PPTs, or Prezi) demonstrating blood flow through the heart.
   - Collaborate with each other while doing your individual drawings. Look stuff up online. *Help* each other. *Ask* each other questions. *Teach* each other.
   - Student drawings will be turned in to the instructor/TA for grading.
   - Each Team will then utilize a full sheet of paper collaborating to draw a detailed graphic of blood flow through the heart. Or produce a digital presentation (Google Slides, PPTs, or Prezi) demonstrating blood flow through the heart.
5. Randomly selected (roll of the dice) Lab Teams will lead a class discussion of their graphic.
   - Teams will be prepared to do Q&A with students and instructor.
   - All Teams will take a picture of their graphic and electronically submit it to instructor/TA.
   - Each Team will turn in one Team Worksheet to instructor/TA.
6. Instructor will complete "Major Takeaways" with the class.

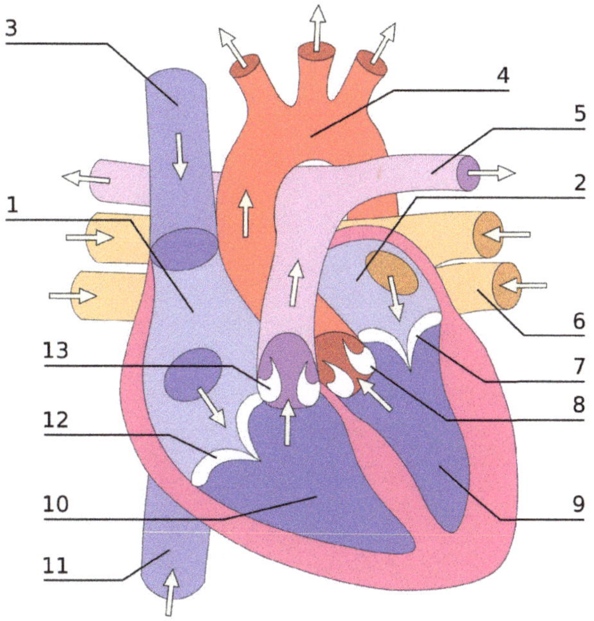

FIGURE 20.1 Label and trace the heart.

Label all thirteen structures and review blood flow through the heart.

Lab Team Worksheet

LAB 20—BLOOD FLOW THROUGH THE HEART/BLOOD TURBULENCE

Team Name: **Date:**

Team members present for Lab:

1.

2.

3.

4.

Collaborating as a Team, answer the following questions. Each Team will turn in *one* Lab Team Worksheet at the completion of Lab.

1. The ______________ valve prevents backflow of blood from the right ventricle into the right atrium.

2. The ____________________ valve prevents backflow of blood from the aorta into the left ventricle.

3. The ________________________________ is known as the heart "pacemaker."

4. A mid-systolic murmur indicates the presence of ________________________.

5. List the three vessels that drain deoxygenated blood into the right atrium.

   ____

   ____

   ____

6. The pulmonary trunk is the outflow tract from the ________________________, carrying blood to the ________________________.

7. The ________________________ drains venous blood from the myocardium into the right atrium.

Figure Credit

Fig. 20.1: Copyright © by Wapcaplet (CC BY-SA 3.0) at https://commons.wikimedia.org/wiki/File:Heart_numlabels.svg.

LAB 21

CVS—The Cardiac Cycle

Purpose of Lab and Desired Outcomes

Participate in Individual and Lab Team Activities to gain insight and understanding into the following topics:

1. Anatomical structure of the heart and great vessels
2. Electrical stimulation of the heart
3. Definition of the cardiac cycle (CC)
4. Details of the cardiac cycle (CC)
5. Pressure gradients and valvular function

Pre-Lab Worksheet

LAB 21—CARDIAC CYCLE

Name: **Date:**

Complete reading assignments for this lab and then answer the following questions:

1. The CVS is the body's ____________________ system.

2. A transportation system has three main divisions. What are they?

   ____

   ____

   ____

3. The ____________________ is the CVS engine providing energy to move blood.

4. The ____________________ demonstrates all the events occurring during a single heartbeat.

5. The cardiac cycle (CC) consists of ____________________ superimposed graphs.

6. The EKG is a graph of ____________________ activity of the heart.

7. The ____________________ is the "pacemaker" of the heart.

8. Both S3 and S4 are caused by ____________________.

In-Lab Activities

1. Collection of student Pre-Lab Worksheets.
2. Instructor calls for QCs (Student Questions, Concerns, Confusions, and need for Clarification).
3. Instructor explanation of In-Lab Activities and desired outcomes from Lab time.
4. Follow the bullet points below to gain insight into the cardiac cycle.
   - Utilizing a blank sheet of standard notebook paper, each Lab Team member will draw a graphic of the cardiac cycle (CC). This must be done in a picture format and not just a copy of the six graphs making up the CC. Be creative! Explain the CC in a picture! Or produce a digital presentation (Google Slides, PPTs, or Prezi) demonstrating the cardiac cycle.
   - Collaborate with each other while doing your drawings. Look stuff up online. *Help* each other. *Ask* each other questions. *Teach* each other.
   - Student drawings will be turned in to the instructor/TA for grading.
   - Each Team will then utilize a large sheet of paper and collaborate to draw a detailed graphic picture of the CC. Or produce a digital presentation (Google Slides, PPTs, or Prezi) demonstrating the cardiac cycle.
5. Randomly selected (roll of the dice) Lab Teams will lead a class discussion of their graphic.
   - Teams will be prepared to do Q&A with students and instructor.
   - All Teams will take a picture of their graphics and electronically submit it to instructor/TA.
   - Each Team will turn in one Team Worksheet to instructor/TA.
6. Instructor will complete "Major Takeaways" with the class.

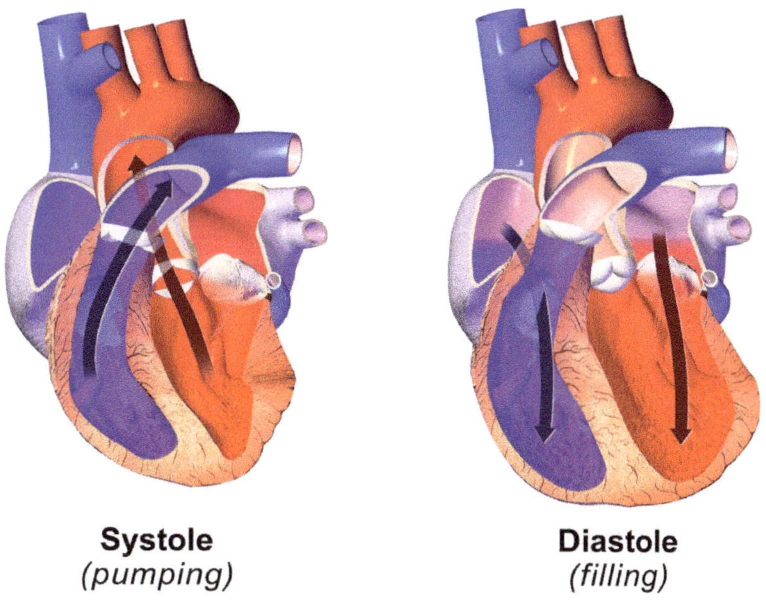

FIGURE 21.1 Diastolic and systolic phases in the cardiac cycle. Simplistic graphic demonstrating ventricular contraction and relaxation.

Lab Team Worksheet

LAB 21—CARDIAC CYCLE

Team Name: **Date:**

Team members present for Lab:

1.

2.

3.

4.

Collaborating as a Team, answer the following questions. Each Team will turn in *one* Lab Team Worksheet at the completion of Lab.

1. Fluids, like blood, flow from areas of higher to lower ________________.

2. The ________________ valve ________________ when the pressure in the left atrium exceeds the pressure in the left ventricle.

3. The ________________ valve ________________ when the pressure in the left ventricle exceeds the pressure in the aorta.

4. The ________________ valve ________________ when the pressure in the left ventricle drops below the pressure in the aorta.

5. The ________________ valve ________________ when the pressure in the left ventricle drops below the pressure in the left atrium.

6. The QRS complex in the EKQ shows ________________ depolarization.

Figure Credit

LAB 22

Immune System—Blood Typing

Purpose of Lab and Desired Outcomes

Participate in Individual and Lab Team Activities to gain insight and understanding into the following topics:

1. Composition of blood
2. Innate immunity
3. Adaptive immunity
4. Blood typing as an example of adaptive immunity

Pre-Lab Worksheet

LAB 22—IMMUNE SYSTEM—BLOOD TYPING

Name: **Date:**

Each student will answer the following questions *before* coming to Lab.
Complete the reading assignment for this lab and then answer the following questions. The CVS Flow Chart (Figure 14.1 in *SS A&P* text, 2nd Edition) will be helpful as well as the H_2O Sheet.

1. The cardiovascular system (CVS) is the body's transportation system. What represents the "vehicles" in the CVS?

   ____

2. Blood has two components. What are they?

   ____

   ____

3. Blood is which of the four primary tissue types? ______________________________

4. List the two divisions of the immune system.

   ____

   ____

5. The adaptive immune system differentiates ____________________ from ____________________.

6. Antigens are what type of biochemical (C, P, L, N)? ______________________________

7. Cell surface ______________________________ act as identifying molecules, which the adaptive immune system uses to differentiate self from non-self.

In-Lab Activities

1. Collection of student Pre-Lab Worksheets.
2. Instructor calls for QCs (Student Questions, Concerns, Confusions, and need for Clarification).
3. Instructor explanation of In-Lab Activities and desired outcomes from Lab time.
4. Follow the bullet points below to gain insight into blood typing and adaptive immunity.
   - Utilizing a blank sheet of standard notebook paper, each Lab Team member will draw a graphic of blood typing. This must be done in a picture format. Utilize Figure 15.1 in *SS A&P,* 2nd Edition, and be creative! How does blood typing demonstrate adaptive immunity? Or produce a digital presentation (Google Slides, PPTs, or Prezi) demonstrating blood typing.
   - Collaborate with each other while doing your individual drawings. Look stuff up online. *Help* each other. *Ask* each other questions. *Teach* each other.
   - Student drawings will be turned in to the instructor/TA for grading.
   - Each Team will then utilize a large sheet of paper collaborating to draw a detailed graphic picture explaining blood typing, including surface antigens and host antibodies. Or produce a digital presentation (Google Slides, PPTs, or Prezi) demonstrating blood typing.
5. Randomly selected (roll of the dice) Lab Teams will lead a class discussion of their graphic.
   - Teams will be prepared to do Q&A with students and instructor.
   - All Teams will take a picture of their graphics and electronically submit it to instructor/TA.
   - Each Team will turn in one Team Worksheet to instructor/TA.
6. Instructor will complete "Major Takeaways" with the class.

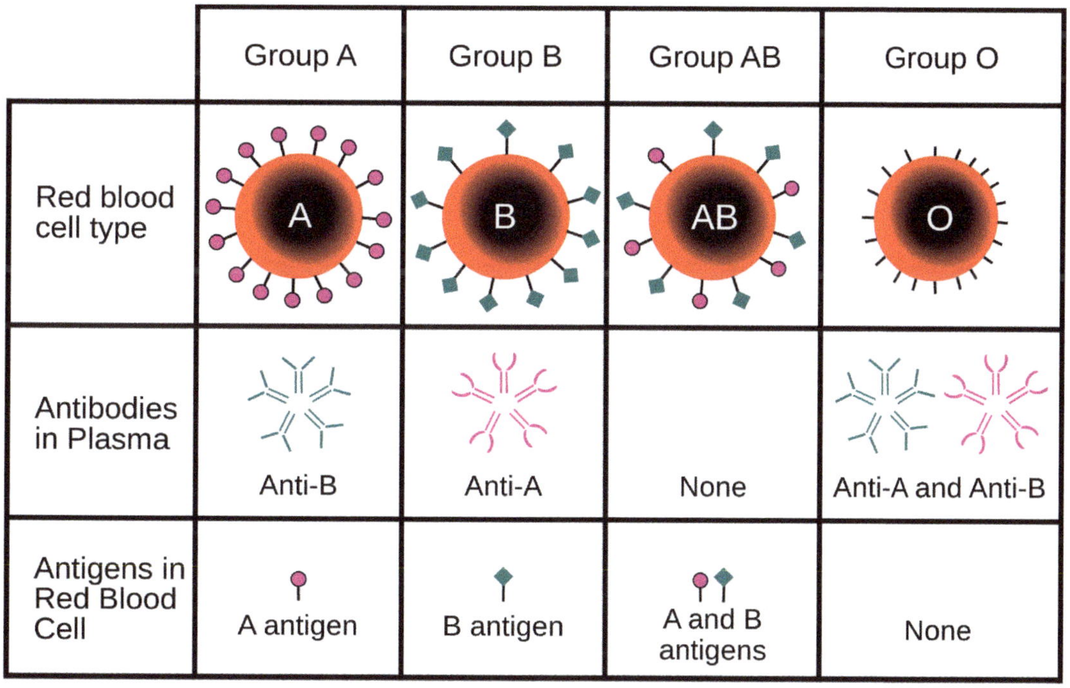

FIGURE 22.1 Chart summary of ABO blood typing antigens and antibodies. Simplistic graphic demonstrating the presence of antigens and antibodies in blood typing.

Lab Team Worksheet

LAB 22—IMMUNE SYSTEM—BLOOD TYPING

Team Name: **Date:**

Team members present for Lab:

1.

2.

3.

4.

Collaborating as a Team, answer the following questions. Each Team will turn in *one* Lab Team Worksheet at the completion of Lab.

1. The adaptive immune system differentiates ____________________ from ____________________.

2. Cell surface ____________________ are ____________________ molecules, which act like the "fingerprints" on the cell surface of red blood cells (RBCs).

3. A person with AB^+ type blood has how many surface antigens on its RBCs? ____________________

4. List the cell surface antigens on the surface of RBCs in a person with AB^+ type blood.

    ____

    ____

    ____

5. A person with O^- blood has how many surface antigens on its RBCs? ____________________

6. A person with ____________________ type blood can safely donate blood to any other blood type.

Figure Credit

Fig. 22.1: Source: https://commons.wikimedia.org/wiki/File:ABO_blood_type.svg.

LAB 23

Immune and Lymphatic Systems

Purpose of Lab and Desired Outcomes

Participate in Individual and Lab Team Activities to gain insight and understanding into the following topics:

1. Anatomical structure of the lymphatic system
2. Interstitial fluid (two primary fluid compartments)
3. Immune system—innate and adaptive (acquired)
4. Barrier and non-barrier defense
5. Antigen-antibody interactions

Pre-Lab Worksheet

LAB 23—IMMUNE AND LYMPHATIC SYSTEMS

Name: **Date:**

Each student will answer the following questions before coming to Lab.
Complete the reading assignments for this lab. Then, answer the following questions:

1. The immune system is the body's ______________________ system.

2. List the two divisions of the immune system.

____

____

3. The lymphatic system drains ______________________ fluid into the CVS.

4. The ________________ ________________ ________________ drains lymph from the right upper extremity, the right half of the thoracic region, and the right half of the head and neck.

5. Most of the body's lymph is drained into the CVS by the ______________________.

6. List the two divisions of the innate immune system.

____

____

7. List one example of a non-barrier type of innate immunity.

____

In-Lab Activities

1. Collection of student Pre-Lab Worksheets.
2. Instructor calls for QCs (Student Questions, Concerns, Confusions, and need for Clarification).
3. Instructor explanation of In-Lab Activities and desired outcomes from Lab time.
4. Follow the bullet points below to gain insight into immunity and the lymphatic system.
   - Utilizing a blank sheet of standard notebook paper, each Lab Team member will draw a conceptual diagram of the immune system, including both innate and adaptive divisions. This must be done in a picture format. Be creative! Or produce a digital presentation (Google Slides, PPTs, or Prezi) demonstrating the immune system.
   - Collaborate with each other while doing your individual drawings. Look stuff up online. *Help* each other. *Ask* each other questions. *Teach* each other! Or produce a digital presentation (Google Slides, PPTs, or Prezi) demonstrating the immune system.
   - Student drawings will be turned in to the instructor/TA for evaluation.
   - Each Team will then utilize a large sheet of paper collaborating to draw a detailed graphic picture explaining immunity, including both innate (barrier/non-barrier) and adaptive (antigen/antibody reaction). Or produce a digital presentation (Google Slides, PPTs, or Prezi) demonstrating the immune system.
5. Randomly selected (roll of the dice) Lab Teams will lead a discussion of their graphic with the class.
   - Teams will be prepared to do Q&A with students and instructor.
   - All Teams will take a picture of their graphics and electronically submit it to instructor/TA.
   - Each Team will turn in one Team Worksheet to instructor/TA.
6. Instructor will complete "Major Takeaways" with the class.

Lab Team Worksheet

LAB 23—IMMUNE AND LYMPHATIC SYSTEMS

Team Name: **Date:**

Team members present for Lab:

1.

2.

3.

4.

Collaborating as a Team, answer the following questions. Each Team will turn in *one* Lab Team Worksheet at the completion of Lab.

1. List the two major components that make up lymph.

____

____

2. List three examples of non-barrier innate immunity.

____

____

____

3. The presence of ________________ allow the immune system to differentiate self from non-self.

4. List the two divisions of the adaptive immune system.

____

____

5. A vaccination is an example of ________________ ________________ immunity.

6. Breast milk provides the baby with ________________ ________________ immunity.

LAB 24

Respiratory System—Anatomy

Purpose of Lab and Desired Outcomes

Participate in Individual and Lab Team Activities to gain insight and understanding into the following topics:

1. Structure of the respiratory system
2. Function of the respiratory system
3. Conducting zone and the respiratory zone
4. Epithelial tissues lining the respiratory system
5. Muscles of breathing

Pre-Lab Worksheet

LAB 24—RESPIRATORY SYSTEM—ANATOMY

Name: **Date:**

Each student will answer the following questions *before* coming to Lab.
Complete the reading assignments for this Lab Activity. Then, answer the following questions. The H_2O Sheet will help! (Figure 2.1 in *SS A&P* text, 2nd Edition.)

1. The primary function of the respiratory system is ____________________________.

2. What are the two zones of the respiratory system?

____

____

3. The specific tissue lining the large bronchi of the lungs is ____________________________.

4. The specific tissue lining the alveolar sacs is ____________________________.

5. The alveoli are ____________________ the way they are because of what they ____________________.

6. The ____________________________ is the major muscle of breathing.

7. List the two primary gases that are exchanged in the lungs.

____

____

In-Lab Activities

1. Collection of student Pre-Lab Worksheets.
2. Instructor calls for QCs (Student Questions, Concerns, Confusions, and need for Clarification).
3. Instructor explanation of In-Lab Activities and desired outcomes from Lab time.
4. Utilizing anatomical models, online resources, and pictures, student Teams will work collaboratively to identify the following structures of the respiratory system.

Major structures of the respiratory system—students need to be able to "run" or trace the respiratory tract from nares to alveoli.

- Lungs
    - Left
        - Two lobes
        - One fissure
        - Cardiac notch
    - Right
        - Three lobes
        - Two fissures
    - Hilum—entry/exit area for bronchi, arteries, and veins
- **Conducting zone**
    - Nares or nostrils
    - Nasal cavity with conchae
        - Superior
        - Middle
        - Inferior
    - Pharynx
        - Nasal
        - Oral
        - Laryngeal
    - Larynx
        - True vocal cords
        - False vocal cords
    - Trachea
    - Carina
    - Main stem bronchi
        - Left
        - Right
    - Left and right secondary bronchi
    - Left and right tertiary bronchi
    - Terminal bronchioles
- **Respiratory zone**
    - Respiratory bronchioles
    - Alveolar ducts
    - Alveolar sacs

- **Muscles of breathing**
  - Diaphragm—***major muscle of breathing***
    - Esophageal hiatus
    - Inferior vena cava hiatus
  - Intercostal muscles
    - Internal—expiration
    - External—inspiration
- **Paranasal sinuses**
  - Frontal
  - Ethmoidal
  - Sphenoidal
  - Maxillary
- **Epithelium of the respiratory system**
  - Pseudostratified ciliated columnar epithelium with goblet cells
    - Lines much of the conducting zone—especially larger bronchi
    - Nasal cavity
    - Nasopharynx
    - Paranasal sinuses
    - Trachea
    - Inferior portion of larynx
    - Main stem bronchi
    - Lobar bronchi
  - Simple ciliated columnar epithelium
    - Segmental bronchi
    - Large bronchioles
  - Simple ciliated cuboid epithelium
    - Terminal bronchioles
    - Respiratory bronchioles
  - Simple squamous epithelium
    - Alveolar ducts
    - Alveolar sacs

While working to identify the above structures, Teams will concurrently do the following:

- On a large sheet of paper, draw out a *conceptual graphic* of the respiratory tract—both conducting and respiratory zones. Or produce a digital presentation (Google Slides, PPTs, or Prezi) of a conceptual graphic of the respiratory system.
- On a second large sheet of paper, draw out a conceptual graphic of the four different types of epithelium that line the respiratory tract. Or produce a digital presentation (Google Slides, PPTs, or Prezi) of a conceptual graphic of the four different types of epithelium that line the respiratory system.
- Teams will prepare to explain their graphics during class discussion time in #5.

5. Randomly selected (roll of the dice) Lab Teams will lead a class discussion of their graphics.
   - Teams will be prepared to do Q&A with students and instructor.
   - All Teams will take a picture of their graphics and electronically submit it to instructor/TA.
   - Each Team will turn in one Team Worksheet to instructor/TA.
6. Instructor will complete "Major Takeaways" with the class.

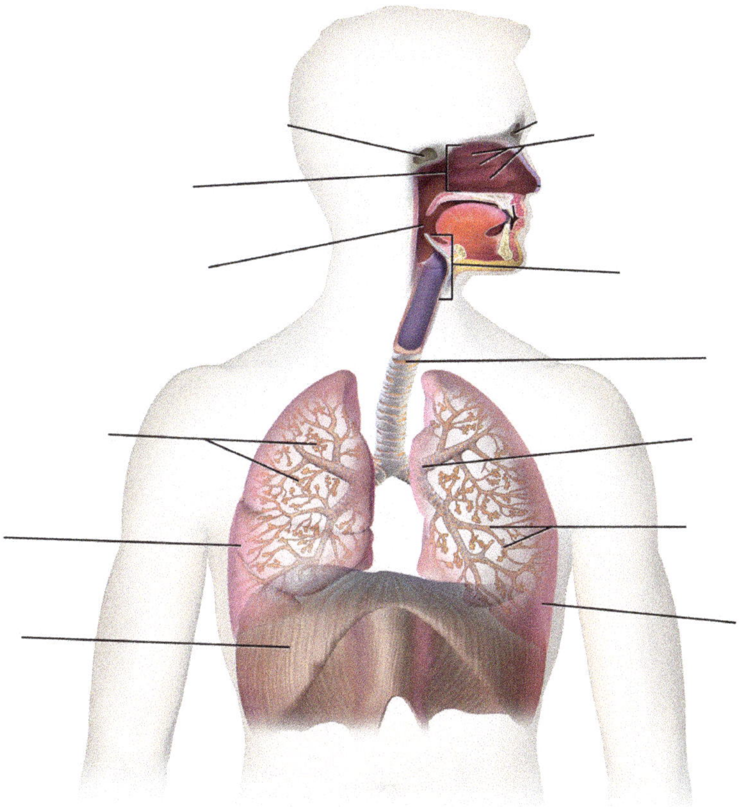

FIGURE 24.1 Labeling opportunity for the respiratory system.

Label the structures of the respiratory tract. What is the difference between the conducting and respiratory zones?

Lab Team Worksheet

LAB 24—RESPIRATORY SYSTEM—ANATOMY

Team Name: **Date:**

Team members present for Lab:

1.

2.

3.

4.

Collaborating as a Team, answer the following questions. Each Team will turn in *one* Lab Team Worksheet at the completion of Lab.

1. The primary function of the respiratory system is ____________ ____________.

2. The alveolar sacs are shaped like bunches of grapes, which increases the internal ____________ ____________, facilitating gas exchange.

3. The lungs exchange ____________ and ____________ ____________.

4. The respiratory and digestive tracts involve two of the same structures. What are they?

   ____

   ____

5. The epithelium lining the alveolar sacs is ____________.

6. Goblet cells produce ____________.

7. The left lung has a depression called the ____________ ____________.

8. The right lung has ____________ lobes.

Figure Credit

LAB 25

Respiratory System (RS) and Ventilation

Purpose of Lab and Desired Outcomes

Participate in Individual and Lab Team Activities to gain insight and understanding into the following topics:

1. Anatomical structure of the respiratory system
2. Boyle's law
3. Muscles of breathing
4. Movement of air into and out of the lungs
5. Gas exchange in the lungs
6. Gas exchange at the tissue level

Pre-Lab Worksheet

LAB 25—RESPIRATORY SYSTEM AND VENTILATION

Name: **Date:**

Each student will answer the following questions *before* coming to Lab.

Complete the reading assignment for this lab activity. Then, answer the following questions. As always, your H_2O Sheet will help. (Figure 2.1 in *SS A&P* text, 2nd Edition.)

1. The conceptual function of the respiratory system is ________________________.

2. List the two gases that are exchanged in the lungs.

____

____

3. The ________________________ are the functional units of the RS.

4. The ________________________ is the major muscle of breathing.

5. List three accessory muscles of breathing, either inspiratory or expiratory.

____

____

____

6. The diaphragm is innervated by what division of the nervous system? ____________________

In-Lab Activities

1. Collection of student Pre-Lab Worksheets.
2. Instructor calls for QCs (Student Questions, Concerns, Confusions, and need for Clarification).
3. Instructor explanation of In-Lab Activities and desired outcomes from Lab time.
4. Follow the bullet points below to gain insight into ventilation and the respiratory system.
   - Utilizing a blank sheet of standard notebook paper, Lab Team members will draw a conceptual diagram of Boyle's law. This must be done in a picture format. Do *not* write out the formula for Boyle's law. Use your imagination! Be creative! Or produce a digital presentation (Google Slides, PPTs, or Prezi) of a conceptual graphic of Boyle's law.
   - Collaborate with each other while doing your individual drawings. Look stuff up online. *Help* each other. *Ask* each other questions. *Teach* each other.
   - Student drawings will be turned in to the instructor/TA for grading.
   - Each Team will then utilize a large sheet of paper collaborating to draw a detailed graphic explaining Boyle's law. Or produce a digital presentation (Google Slides, PPTs, or Prezi) of a conceptual graphic of Boyle's law.
   - On a second large sheet of paper, Teams will collaborate to draw a conceptual flow chart showing gas exchange in the lungs on the top half of the sheet and at the tissue level on the bottom half of the sheet. Or produce a digital presentation (Google Slides, PPTs, or Prezi) of a conceptual graphic showing gas exchange in the lungs and tissues.
5. Randomly selected (roll of the dice) Lab Teams will lead a class discussion of their graphics.
   - Teams will be prepared to do Q&A with students and instructor.
   - All Teams will take a picture of their graphics and electronically submit it to instructor/TA.
   - Each Team will turn in one Team Worksheet to instructor/TA.
6. Instructor will complete "Major Takeaways" with the class.

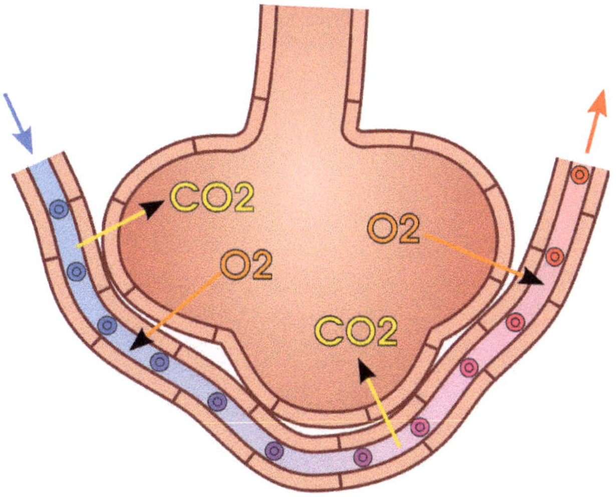

FIGURE 25.1 Simplistic graphic of basic lung function—gas exchange. Simplistic graphic showing gas exchange in an alveolar sac.

Lab Team Worksheet

LAB 25—RESPIRATORY SYSTEM AND VENTILATION

Team Name: **Date:**

Team members present for Lab:

1.

2.

3.

4.

Collaborating as a Team, answer the following questions. Each Team will turn in *one* Lab Team Worksheet at the completion of Lab.

1. When the diaphragm contracts the ________________ of the pleural cavities ________________.

2. When the diaphragm relaxes the ________________ of the pleural cavities ________________.

3. When the diaphragm contracts, air moves ______________________________ the lungs.

4. When the diaphragm relaxes, air moves ______________________________ the lungs.

5. Boyle's law states that in a closed container filled with a gas, the pressure and volume are ______________________________ related.

6. The amount of air moving in and out of the lungs while at rest is the ________________________ volume.

7. ______________ capacity is the amount of air that can be fully expired after a maximum inhalation.

8. The majority of CO_2 produced by cellular metabolism is transported to the lungs by combining with water to form ______________________________ acid.

Figure Credit

LAB 26

Digestive System—Nutrient Breakdown

Purpose of Lab and Desired Outcomes

Participate in individual and Lab Team Activities to gain insight and understanding into the following topics:

1. The conceptual function of the digestive system
2. The three primary sources of nutrition
3. The gastric pit—structure and function
4. Phases of gastrointestinal digestion
5. Regulation of digestion and nutrient absorption
6. Ability to "run" GI tract

Pre-Lab Worksheet

LAB 26—DIGESTIVE SYSTEM—NUTRIENT BREAKDOWN

Name: **Date:**

Each student will answer the following questions *before* coming to Lab.

Complete the reading assignments for this lab activity. Then, answer the following questions. As always, your H_2O Sheet will help.

1. According to the H_2O Sheet, the conceptual function of the digestive system provides two things. What are they?

 ____

 ____

2. List the two divisions of the digestive system.

 ____

 ____

3. What are the three distinguishing anatomical characteristics of the small intestine?

 ____

 ____

 ____

4. The initials that indicate the three primary sources of nutrition are ______________.

5. The primary source of glucose is ______________.

6. Proteins break down into smaller units called ______________ ______________.

In-Lab Activities

1. Collection of student Pre-Lab Worksheets.
2. Instructor calls for QCs (Student Questions, Concerns, Confusions, and need for Clarification).
3. Instructor explanation of In-Lab Activities and desired outcomes from Lab time.
4. Follow the bullet points below to gain insight into digestion.
    - Utilizing a blank sheet of standard notebook paper, each Lab Team member will draw a conceptual diagram explaining the gastric pit, including the three primary cells, their secretions, and how those secretions interact to facilitate digestion in the stomach. Use your imagination! Explain gastric pits in pictures. Be creative! Or produce a digital presentation (Google Slides, PPTs, or Prezi) of conceptual graphics explaining gastric pits.
    - Collaborate with each other while doing your individual drawings. Look stuff up online. *Help* each other. *Ask* each other questions. *Teach* each other.
    - Student drawings will be turned in to the instructor/TA for grading.
    - Each Team will then utilize a large sheet of paper collaborating to draw a detailed graphic explaining the gastric pit. Or produce a digital presentation (Google Slides, PPTs, or Prezi) of conceptual graphics explaining gastric pits.
    - On a second large sheet of paper, Teams will collaborate to draw a conceptual flow chart of the three phases of gastrointestinal digestion. Teams will be prepared to discuss both graphics with the class. Or produce a digital presentation (Google Slides, PPTs, or Prezi) of conceptual graphics explaining the three phases of gastrointestinal digestion.
5. Randomly selected (roll of the dice) Lab Teams will lead a class discussion of their graphic.
    - Teams will be prepared to do Q&A with students and instructor.
    - All Teams will take a picture of their graphics and electronically submit it to instructor/TA.
    - Each Team will turn in one Team Worksheet to instructor/TA.
6. Instructor will complete "Major Takeaways" with the class.

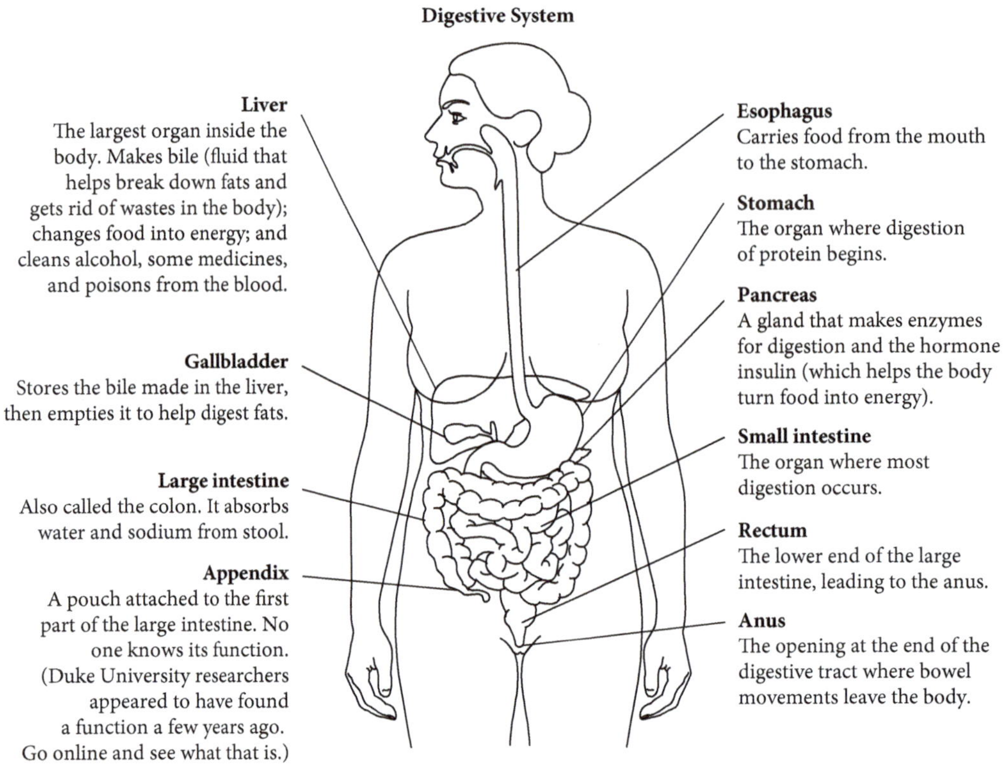

FIGURE 26.1 Super Simple diagram showing major structures and functions of DS.

Write out a list of *all* the structures of the digestive system. What is the function of each? This needs to be a detailed list including sphincters, parts of the small intestine, flexures, and parts of the large intestine. Students need to be able to "run" or trace the GI tract from mouth and oral cavity to anal canal and anus.

Lab Team Worksheet

LAB 26—DIGESTIVE SYSTEM—NUTRIENT BREAKDOWN

Team Name: **Date:**

Team members present for Lab:

1.

2.

3.

4.

Collaborating as a Team, answer the following questions. Each Team will turn in *one* Lab Team Worksheet at the completion of Lab.

1. List the three phases of swallowing.

 ____

 ____

 ____

2. The ______________________ phase of swallowing is when the food bolus is voluntarily pushed by the tongue against the hard palate toward the oropharynx.

3. The esophageal phase of swallowing involves ______________________ muscle, which is innervated by ______________________ neurons.

4. Parietal cells in the gastric pits produce ______________________ and ______________________.

5. The chief cells in the gastric pits produce pepsinogen, a precursor to ______________________.

6. The ______________________ has a dual endocrine/exocrine function, including the secretion of all three of the digestive enzymes: amylase, protease, and lipase.

Figure Credit

Fig. 26.1: Source: https://commons.wikimedia.org/wiki/File:Gastrointestinal_system.gif.

LAB 27

Urinary System—Anatomy

Purpose of Lab and Desired Outcomes

Participate in Individual and Lab Team Activities to gain insight and understanding into the following topics:

1. Structure of the urinary system
2. Structure of the nephron

Pre-Lab Worksheet

LAB 27—URINARY SYSTEM—ANATOMY

Name: **Date:**

Each student will answer the following questions *before* coming to Lab.
Complete the reading assignments for this Lab Activity. Then, answer the following questions. The H_2O Sheet will help! (Figure 2.1 in *SS A&P* text, 2nd Edition.)

1. The primary function of the urinary system is to ______________________ and

   ______________________.

2. The ______________________ are located in a retroperitoneal location.

3. The specific tissue that lines the urinary bladder is ______________________.

4. List the four gross structures that make up the urinary system.

   ____

   ____

   ____

   ____

5. The urinary system filters waste from the ______________________.

6. The major muscle of the urinary bladder is the ______________________ muscle.

In-Lab Activities

1. Collection of student Pre-Lab Worksheets.
2. Instructor calls for QCs (Student Questions, Concerns, Confusions, and need for Clarification).
3. Instructor explanation of In-Lab Activities and desired outcomes from lab time.
4. Utilizing anatomical models, online resources, and pictures, student Teams will work collaboratively to identify the following structures of the urinary system.

Major Structures of the Urinary System

- **Gross urinary structures**—able to "run" renal structures from kidney through urethra
  - Kidneys—left and right—retroperitoneal (What's that mean?)
  - Ureters
    - Left
    - Right
  - Urinary bladder
  - Urethra
- **Gross kidney anatomy—frontal section**
  - Areas
    - Cortex
    - Medulla
  - Renal column
  - Renal pyramid
  - Renal papillae
  - Renal pelvis
  - Minor calyx
  - Major calyx
  - Renal capsule
  - Renal artery
  - Renal vein
- **Nephron and internal renal structures—microscopic anatomy**
  - CVS—contribution to nephron
    - Afferent arteriole
    - Efferent arteriole
  - Renal corpuscle
    - Glomerulus
    - Glomerular capsule—Bowman's capsule
  - Proximal convoluted tubule
  - Loop of Henle
    - Descending limb
    - Ascending limb
  - Distal convoluted tubule
  - Juxtaglomerular apparatus

- Collecting duct
- Renal papillae

While working to identify the above structures, Teams will concurrently do the following:

- On a large sheet of paper, draw out a graphic of the gross urinary structures—kidneys, ureters, urinary bladder, and urethra. Or produce a digital presentation (Google Slides, PPTs, or Prezi) of a conceptual graphic demonstrating the gross structures of the urinary system.
- On a second large sheet of paper, Teams will draw out the nephron structure starting with the afferent and efferent arterioles and the renal corpuscle through the collecting duct. Or produce a digital presentation (Google Slides, PPTs, or Prezi) of the nephron structure.
- Teams will prepare to explain their graphics during class discussion time in #5 below.

5. Randomly selected (roll of the dice) Lab Teams will lead a class discussion of their graphics.
    - Teams will be prepared to do Q&A with students and instructor.
    - All Teams will take a picture of their graphics and electronically submit it to instructor/TA.
    - Each Team will turn in one Team Worksheet to instructor/TA.
6. Instructor will complete "Major Takeaways" with the class.

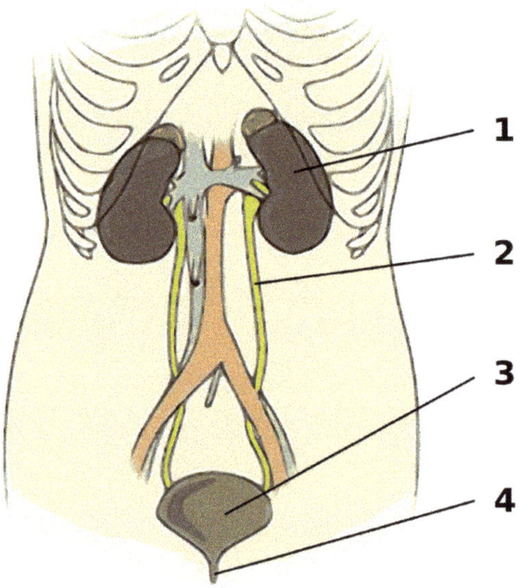

FIGURE 27.1 Urinary system.

Label the four major structures of the urinary system.

Lab Team Worksheet

LAB 27 URINARY SYSTEM—ANATOMY

Team Name: **Date:**

Team Members present for Lab:

1.

2.

3.

4.

Collaborating as a Team, answer the following questions. Each Team will turn in *one* Lab Team Worksheet at the completion of Lab.

1. List the four major gross structures of the urinary system.

____

____

____

____

2. The production of urine requires an interface between two systems. What are they?

____

____

3. The kidney is in a ______________ position, located behind the peritoneum.

4. The urinary bladder is ______________ the way it is because of what it ______________.

5. The tubular structure running from the urinary bladder to outside the body is called the ______________.

Figure Credit

Fig. 27.1: Source: https://commons.wikimedia.org/wiki/File:Illu_urinary_system_numbers.svg.

LAB 28

Urinary System—Physiology

Purpose of Lab and Desired Outcomes

Participate in Individual and Lab Team Activities to gain insight and understanding into the following topics:

1. Anatomical structure of the urinary system
2. The nephron: functional and structural unit of the kidney
3. Conceptual function of the urinary system

Pre-Lab Worksheet

LAB 28—URINARY SYSTEM—PHYSIOLOGY

Name: **Date:**

Each student will answer the following questions *before* coming to Lab.

Complete the reading assignment for this activity. Then, answer the following questions. As always, your H_2O Sheet will help.

1. According to the H_2O Sheet, the urinary system filters ______________________ from the blood and ______________________ "stuff."

2. The structural and functional unit of the urinary system is the ______________________.

3. List the three phases of urine formation.

____

____

____

4. The kidneys filter approximately ______________ liters of liquid every twenty-four hours from the blood.

5. Average urine production is ______________ to ______________ liters per day.

6. Most of the liquid filtered into the glomerular space is ______________________ by the cells lining the kidney tubules.

In-Lab Activities

1. Collection of student Pre-Lab Worksheets.
2. Instructor calls for QCs (Student Questions, Concerns, Confusions, and need for Clarification).
3. Instructor explanation of In-Lab Activities and desired outcomes from Lab time.
4. Follow the bullet points below to gain insight into the function of the renal system.
   - Utilizing a blank sheet of standard notebook paper, each Lab Team member will draw a conceptual diagram of how the kidneys function. This can be done in any graphic format the student prefers. In other words, draw a picture showing how the kidneys make urine. Use your imagination! Be creative! Or produce a digital presentation (Google Slides, PPTs, or Prezi) of conceptual graphics explaining kidney function.
   - Collaborate with each other while doing your individual drawings. Look stuff up online. *Help* each other. *Ask* each other questions. *Teach* each other.
   - Student drawings will be turned in to the instructor/TA for grading.
   - Each Team will then utilize a large sheet of paper collaborating to draw a conceptual diagram of how the kidneys function. Or produce a digital presentation (Google Slides, PPTs, or Prezi) of conceptual graphics explaining kidney function.
5. Randomly selected (roll of the dice) Lab Teams will lead a class discussion of their graphic.
   - Teams will be prepared to do Q&A with students and instructor.
   - All Teams will take a picture of their graphics and electronically submit it to instructor/TA.
   - Each Team will turn in one Team Worksheet to instructor/TA.
6. Instructor will complete "Major Takeaways" with the class.

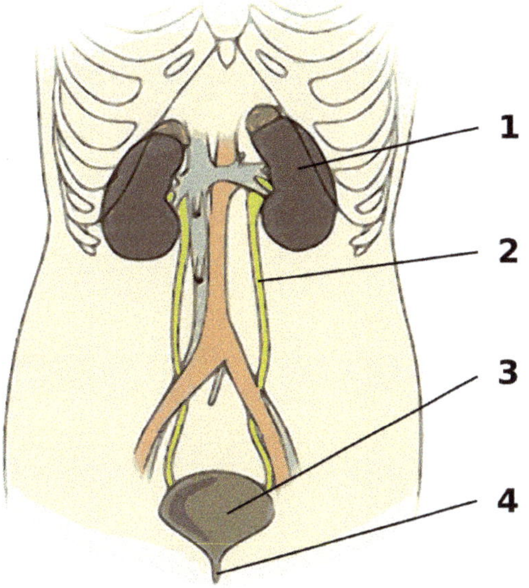

FIGURE 28.1 Label each structure *and* list its function.

What are the functions of the four major organs of the urinary system?

Lab Team Worksheet

LAB 28—URINARY SYSTEM—WASTE AND BALANCE

Team Name: **Date:**

Team members present for Lab:

1.

2.

3.

4.

Collaborating as a Team, answer the following questions. Each Team will turn in *one* Lab Team Worksheet at the completion of Lab.

1. List the three processes of urine formation.

____

____

____

2. List the three opposing forces that create the pressure causing fluid to be forced into the glomerulus.

____

____

____

3. The standard measurement of the amount of filtrate created in one minute is the

____________________.

4. GFR is the abbreviation for ____________________.

5. List two substances that are completely reabsorbed in the PCT.

____

____

Figure Credit

Fig. 28.1: Source: https://commons.wikimedia.org/wiki/File:Illu_urinary_system_numbers.png.

LAB 29

Reproductive System—Anatomy and Physiology

Purpose of Lab and Desired Outcomes

Participate in Individual and Lab Team Activities to gain insight and understanding into the following topics:

1. Structure of the female reproductive system (major organs)
2. Structure of the male reproductive system (major organs)
3. Similarities and differences of the female and male reproductive systems
4. Conceptual function of male and female reproductive systems

Pre-Lab Worksheet

LAB 29—REPRODUCTIVE SYSTEM—ANATOMY AND PHYSIOLOGY

Name: **Date:**

Each student will answer the following questions *before* coming to Lab.
Complete the reading assignments for this Lab Activity. Then answer the following questions. The H_2O Sheet might help! (Figure 2.1 in *SS A&P* text, 2nd Edition.)

1. The primary function of the reproductive system is ______________________.

2. The penis is ______________________ the way it is because of what it ______________________.

3. The specific tissue that lines the urinary bladder in both the female and male is ______________________.

4. List the structures that carry sperm from production in the testis to the outside.

____

____

____

____

____

5. The ______________________ is the sex organ of the female.

In-Lab Activities

1. Collection of student Pre-Lab Worksheets.
2. Instructor calls for QCs (Student Questions, Concerns, Confusions, and need for Clarification).
3. Instructor explanation of In-Lab Activities and desired outcomes from Lab time.
4. Utilizing anatomical models, online resources, and pictures, student Teams will work collaboratively to identify the following structures of the female and male reproductive systems:

Major Structures of the Female Reproductive System:

- Fallopian tubes with fimbriae
- Pubic bone
- Clitoris
- Vestibule
- Urethra
- Labia minora
- Labia majora
- Ovary
- Sigmoid colon
- Uterus
- Fornix
- Cervix
- Rectum
- Vagina
- Anus
- Bartholin's gland

Major Structures of the Male Reproductive System:

- Pubic bone
- External urethral sphincter
- Penis
- Corpus cavernosum
- Glans penis
- Foreskin
- Urethral orifice
- Sigmoid colon
- Rectum
- Seminal vesicle
- Ejaculatory duct
- Prostate gland
- Anus
- Vas deferens
- Epididymis
- Testis
- Scrotum

While working to identify the above structures, Teams will concurrently do the following:

- On a large sheet of paper, draw out a graphic of the gross anatomy demonstrated in a midsagittal section of the female. Or produce a digital presentation (Google Slides, PPTs, or Prezi) of a conceptual graphic demonstrating the gross structures of the female anatomy.
- On a second large sheet of paper, draw out a graphic of the gross anatomy demonstrated in a midsagittal section of the male. Or produce a digital presentation (Google Slides, PPTs, or Prezi) of a conceptual graphic demonstrating the gross structures of the male anatomy.
- Finally, Teams will draw a graphic on a large sheet of paper demonstrating hormonal control and fluctuation in both the male and the female.
- Teams will prepare to explain their graphics during class discussion time in #5.

5. Randomly selected (roll of the dice) Lab Teams will lead a class discussion of their graphics.
    - Teams will be prepared to do Q&A with students and instructor.
    - All Teams will take a picture of their graphics and electronically submit it to instructor/TA.
    - Each Team will turn in one Team Worksheet to instructor/TA.
6. Instructor will complete "Major Takeaways" with the class.

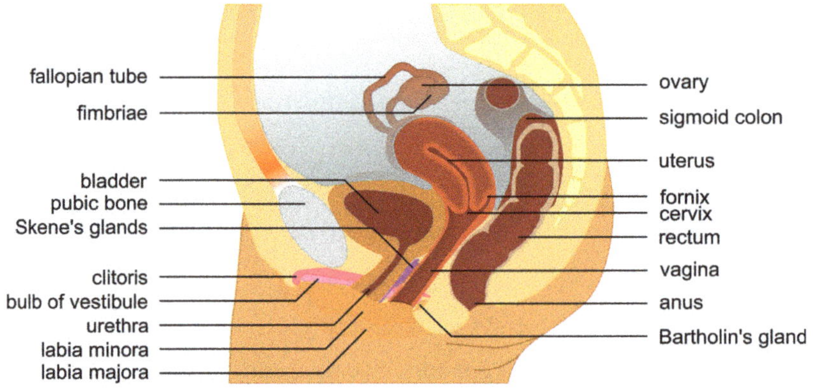

FIGURE 29.1 Midsagittal female pelvis.

Important structures and areas for the novice student.

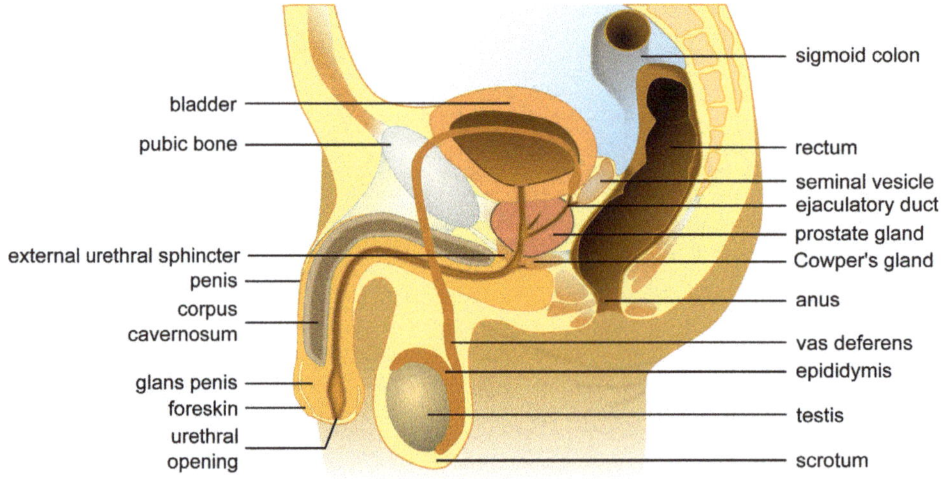

FIGURE 29.2 Midsagittal male pelvis.

Important structures and areas for the novice student.

Lab Team Worksheet

LAB 29—REPRODUCTIVE SYSTEM—ANATOMY AND PHYSIOLOGY

Team Name: **Date:**

Team Members present for Lab:

1.

2.

3.

4.

Collaborating as a Team, answer the following questions. Each Team will turn in *one* Lab Team Worksheet at the completion of Lab.

1. List four structures tracing the path of an oocyte (egg) from the organ of ovulation to the vagina.

____

____

____

____

2. What organs in the female and male have a dual exocrine and endocrine function?

____

____

3. LH and _______________ are the two controlling hormones of the reproductive system.

4. The sex organ of the male is the _______________.

5. The vagina is _______________ the way it is because of what it _______________.

Figure Credits

LAB 30

Nutrition and Metabolism

Purpose of Lab and Desired Outcomes

Participate in individual and Lab Team Activities to gain insight and understanding into the following topics:

1. Nutrition
2. Basic nutrients
3. Lipid transport

Pre-Lab Worksheet

LAB 30—NUTRITION AND METABOLISM

Name: **Date:**

Each student will answer the following questions before coming to Lab.
Complete the reading assignments for this lab activity. Then, answer the following questions:

1. According to the H_2O Sheet, the conceptual function of the digestive system provides two things. What are they?

____

____

2. The study of how living organisms obtain and utilize nutrients is called ______________.

3. What are the four primary biochemical macromolecules involved in human nutrition?

____

____

____

____

4. The majority of the cholesterol in the bloodstream is manufactured in the ______________.

5. Nutrients are divided into what two categories?

____

____

In-Lab Activities

1. Collection of student Pre-Lab Worksheets.
2. Instructor calls for QCs (Student Questions, Concerns, Confusions, and need for Clarification).
3. Instructor explanation of In-Lab Activities and desired outcomes from Lab time.
4. Follow the bullet points below to gain insight into nutrition and metabolism, specifically lipid transport.
    - Each Team will utilize one or more large sheets of paper collaborating to draw a detailed graphic explaining the basic nutrients carbohydrates, proteins, and lipids, including the details of fats (triglycerides, saturated, unsaturated, phospholipids, steroids, and cholesterol). Or produce a digital presentation (Google Slides, PPTs, or Prezi) of a conceptual graphic explaining the basic nutrients.
    - On a second large sheet of paper, Teams will collaborate to draw a conceptual graphic demonstrating the lipoproteins involved in lipid transportation. Or produce a digital presentation (Google Slides, PPTs, or Prezi) of a conceptual graphic explaining the lipoproteins involved in lipid transportation. Teams will be prepared to discuss all graphics with the class.
5. Randomly selected (roll of the dice) Lab Teams will lead a class discussion of their graphic.
    - Teams will be prepared to do Q&A with students and instructor.
    - All Teams will take a picture of their graphics and electronically submit it to instructor/TA.
    - Each Team will turn in one Team Worksheet to instructor/TA.
6. Instructor will complete "Major Takeaways" with the class.

Lab Team Worksheet

LAB 30—NUTRITION AND METABOLISM

Team Name: **Date:**

Team members present for Lab:

1.

2.

3.

4.

Collaborating as a Team, answer the following questions. Each Team will turn in *one* Lab Team Worksheet at the completion of Lab.

1. ____________________ is needed as the basic building block molecule for the steroid hormones.

2. Most ____________________ in the body is synthesized by the liver.

3. Lipids are ____________________ and ____________________ in plasma.

4. ____________________ are necessary for absorption of fats from the small intestine.

5. What are the three categories of lipoproteins?

   ____

   ____

   ____

6. LDL lipoproteins deliver cholesterol to cells that produce ____________________ hormones.

7. What type of lipoprotein helps protect against cardiovascular disease? ____________________

LAB 31

Fluids and Electrolytes

Purpose of Lab and Desired Outcomes

Participate in Individual and Lab Team Activities to gain insight and understanding into the following topics:

1. Primary fluid compartments of the body
2. Divisions of the extracellular fluid compartment
3. Fluid intake and output
4. Hypertonic and hypotonic fluid movement
5. Acid/base balance
6. Buffering

Pre-Lab Worksheet

LAB 31—FLUIDS AND ELECTROLYTES

Name: **Date:**

Each student will answer the following questions *before* coming to Lab.

Complete the reading assignments for this activity. Then, answer the following questions. Figures 20.1 and 20.2 in *SS A&P* text, 2nd Edition will be helpful.

1. ______________________________ accounts for approximately two-thirds of body weight.

2. List the two primary fluid compartments.

   ____

   ____

3. List the two divisions of the extracellular fluid compartment (ECF).

   ____

   ____

4. ______________________________ fluid makes up two-thirds of body fluids.

5. One-third of ECF is made up of ________________________ ________________________.

6. Two-thirds of ECF is made up of ________________________ ________________________.

7. Loss of water, which always occurs regardless of the state of hydration, is called ________________ water loss.

8. ______________________________ is a cellular process that produces water as a waste product.

In-Lab Activities

1. Collection of student Pre-Lab Worksheets.
2. Instructor calls for QCs (Student Questions, Concerns, Confusions, and need for Clarification).
3. Instructor explanation of In-Lab Activities and desired outcomes from Lab time.
4. Follow the bullet points below to gain insight into fluids and electrolytes.
   - Utilizing a blank sheet of standard notebook paper, each Lab Team member will draw a conceptual diagram of fluid intake and fluid output in the human body. This can be done in any graphic format the student prefers. In other words, draw a picture showing how the body takes in water and how it gets rid of water. Use your imagination! Be creative! Or produce a digital presentation (Google Slides, PPTs, or Prezi) of conceptual graphics explaining fluid intake and output.
   - Collaborate with each other while doing your individual drawings. Look stuff up online. *Help* each other. *Ask* each other questions. *Teach* each other.
   - Individual student drawings will be turned in to the instructor/TA for grading.
   - Each Team will then utilize a large sheet of paper collaborating to draw a conceptual diagram of how the body processes water. Or produce a digital presentation (Google Slides, PPTs, or Prezi) of conceptual graphics explaining how the body processes water.
   - On a second large sheet of paper, Teams will collaborate to draw a graphic demonstrating the effect of hypotonic and hypertonic solutions on the movement of water from intravascular space to intracellular space and vice versa. Or produce a digital presentation (Google Slides, PPTs, or Prezi) of conceptual graphics explaining the effects of tonicity on the movement of water.
5. Randomly selected (roll of the dice) Lab Teams will lead a class discussion of their graphics.
   - Teams will be prepared to do Q&A with students and instructor.
   - All Teams will take a picture of their graphics and electronically submit it to instructor/TA.
   - Each Team will turn in one Team Worksheet to instructor/TA.
6. Instructor will complete "Major Takeaways" with the class.

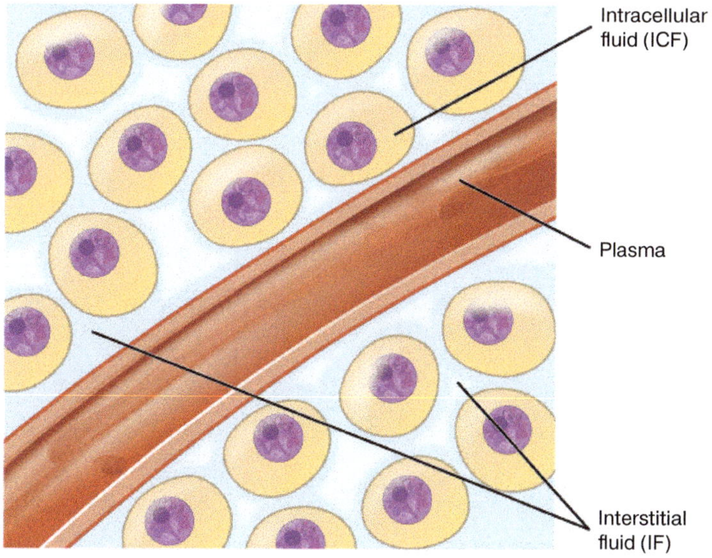

FIGURE 31.1 Super simple graphic showing the three fluid compartments.

Name the fluid compartments in the body. What causes water to move between these compartments?

Lab Team Worksheet

LAB 31—FLUIDS AND ELECTROLYTES

Team Name: **Date:**

Team members present for Lab:

1.

2.

3.

4.

Collaborating as a Team, answer the following questions. Each Team will turn in *one* Lab Team Worksheet at the completion of Lab.

1. List the three fluid compartments.

____

____

____

2. Osmotically active solutes, such as glucose, figuratively "________________" water toward them.

3. The two waste products of CR are ________________________ and carbon dioxide.

4. ________________________ water is the term used to describe the water gained through the food and water we consume.

5. List the four classifications of fluid output.

____

____

____

____

Figure Credit

Fig. 31.1: Copyright © by OpenStax College (CC by 3.0) at https://commons.wikimedia.org/wiki/File:2702_Fluid_Compartments_ICF_ECF.jpg.

LAB 32

Acid/Base Balance and Buffering

Purpose of Lab and Desired Outcomes

Participate in Individual and Lab Team Activities to gain insight and understanding into the following topics:

1. Two primary fluid compartments of the body
2. Divisions of the extracellular fluid compartment
3. Buffer systems
4. Alkalosis and acidosis

Pre-Lab Worksheet

LAB 32—ACID/BASE BALANCE AND BUFFERING

Name: **Date:**

Each student will answer the following questions *before* coming to Lab.

Complete the reading assignments for this lab activity. Then, answer the following questions:

1. ______________________________ accounts for approximately two-thirds of body weight.

2. The body's ability to maintain a relatively constant internal environment is called ______________________________.

3. The acidity of body fluids is measured with the ______________________________ scale.

4. The normal range of plasma pH is ______________________________ to ______________________________.

5. ______________________________ systems help to cushion or balance fluid acidity.

6. List the two types of acid-balancing systems in the body.

   ____

   ____

7. List the two body systems that help to maintain the homeostasis of pH in the body.

   ____

   ____

In-Lab Activities

1. Collection of student Pre-Lab Worksheets.
2. Instructor calls for QCs (Student Questions, Concerns, Confusions, and need for Clarification).
3. Instructor explanation of in-lab activities and desired outcomes from lab time.
4. Follow the bullet points below to gain insight into acid/base balance:
   - Each Team will utilize a large sheet of paper collaborating to write out the complete chemical formula for the bicarbonate buffer system on the top portion of the sheet. Below the formula, Teams will write out the four types of loss of pH balance (acidosis/alkalosis) with one example of a specific cause for each situation. Or produce a digital presentation (Google Slides, PPTs, or Prezi) of conceptual graphics explaining the bicarbonate buffer system and the four types of acidosis/alkalosis.
   - Collaborate with each other while working on the Team graphic. Look stuff up online. *Help* each other. *Ask* each other questions. *Teach* each other.
5. Randomly selected (roll of the dice) Lab Teams will lead a class discussion of their graphic.
   - Teams will be prepared to do Q&A with students and instructor.
   - All Teams will take a picture of their graphics and electronically submit it to instructor/TA.
   - Each Team will turn in one Team Worksheet to instructor/TA.
6. Instructor will complete "Major Takeaways" with the class.

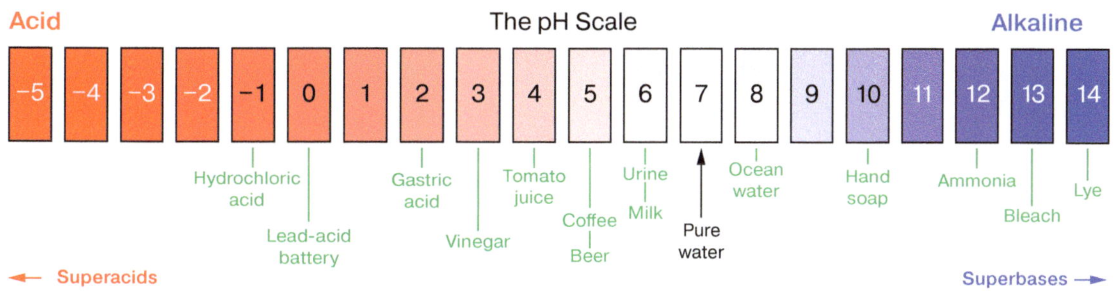

FIGURE 32.1 pH scale with examples of solutions.

What is pH? What causes acidity in the body, and why is it important?

Lab Team Worksheet

LAB 32—ACID/BASE BALANCE AND BUFFERING

Team Name: **Date:**

Team members present for Lab:

1.

2.

3.

4.

Collaborating as a Team, answer the following questions. Each Team will turn in *one* Lab Team Worksheet at the completion of Lab.

1. List the three fluid compartments in the body.

____

____

____

2. List the three specific chemical buffering systems.

____

____

____

3. Write out the chemical formula for the bicarbonate buffer system.

____

4. Excessive use of antacids can cause _______________ alkalosis.

5. Hyperventilation in severe anxiety can cause _______________ alkalosis.

6. Ketoacidosis in diabetes mellitus is one cause of _______________ acidosis.

Figure Credit

Fig. 32.1: Source: https://commons.wikimedia.org/wiki/File:PH_scale_2.png.

CPSIA information can be obtained
at www.ICGtesting.com
Printed in the USA
LVHW060007270522
719862LV00004B/44

9 781793 555694